THE ESSENTIAL Dr. BARBARA COOKBOOK

Unlock 365 Days of Wholesome, Plant-Powered Delights.

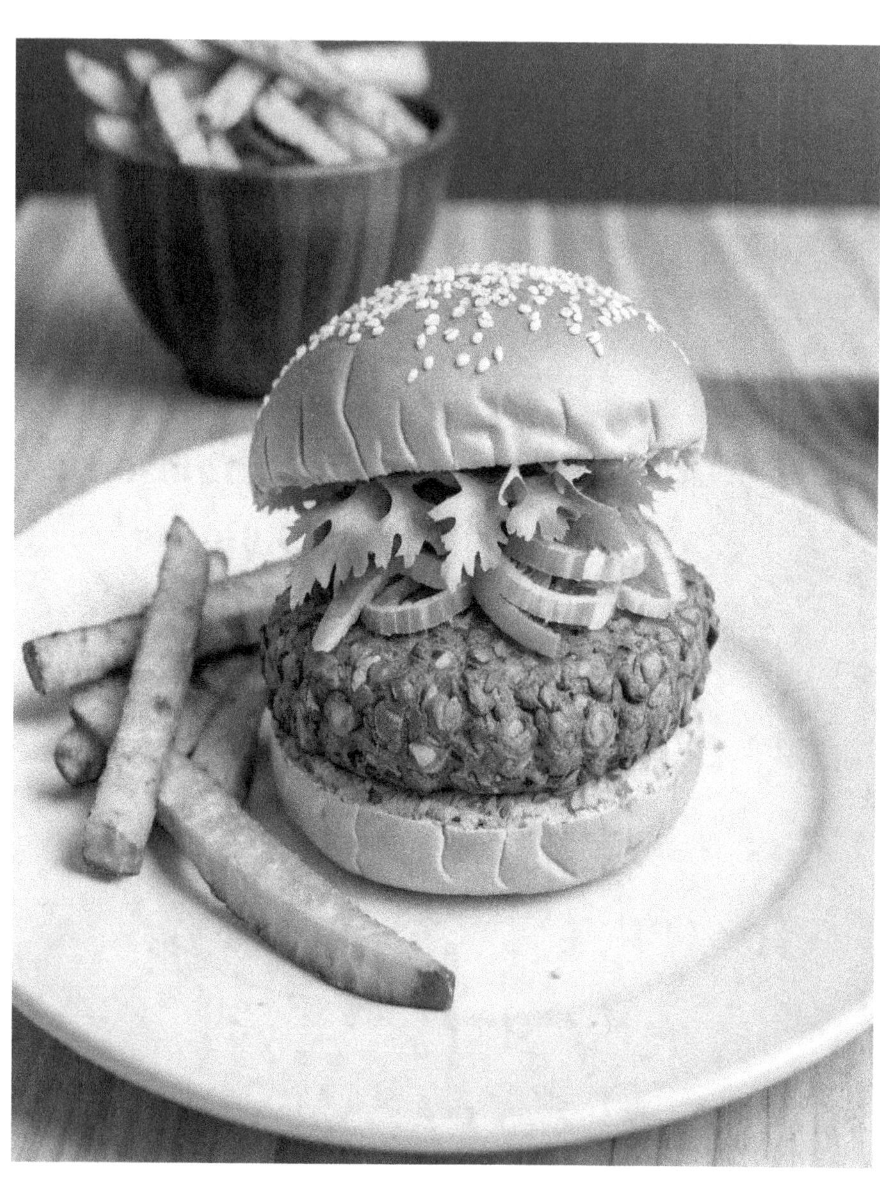

INTRODUCTION

For years, exhaustion was my constant companion. As a busy doctor, I juggled a demanding schedule, relying on convenience foods and caffeine to keep me going. My health suffered. The weight crept on, and I felt a nagging sense of sluggishness. Medication wasn't the answer I craved. Then, I discovered Dr. Barbara O'Neill's revolutionary approach to plant-based nutrition.

It wasn't just about deprivation; it was about a vibrant new way of eating. Skeptical at first, I embarked on a journey of exploration – delving into the wonders of whole grains, colorful vegetables, and legumes. What a transformation! The fog lifted. My energy soared. My body felt lighter, and my taste buds rejoiced in the explosion of flavors.

This cookbook, born from my own experience and inspired by Dr. Barbara's wisdom, is your key to unlocking 365 days of wholesome, plant-powered delights. You won't find bland, restrictive meals here. Instead, discover a treasure trove of delicious recipes that nourish your body and tantalize your palate. Every dish is designed to be easy-to-prepare, perfect for busy lives.

Whether you're a seasoned plant-based chef or just starting your journey, "The Essential Dr. Barbara Cookbook" will be your trusted companion. Let's embark on this adventure together, one delicious bite at a time. You might be surprised by the incredible transformation that awaits you on your plate.

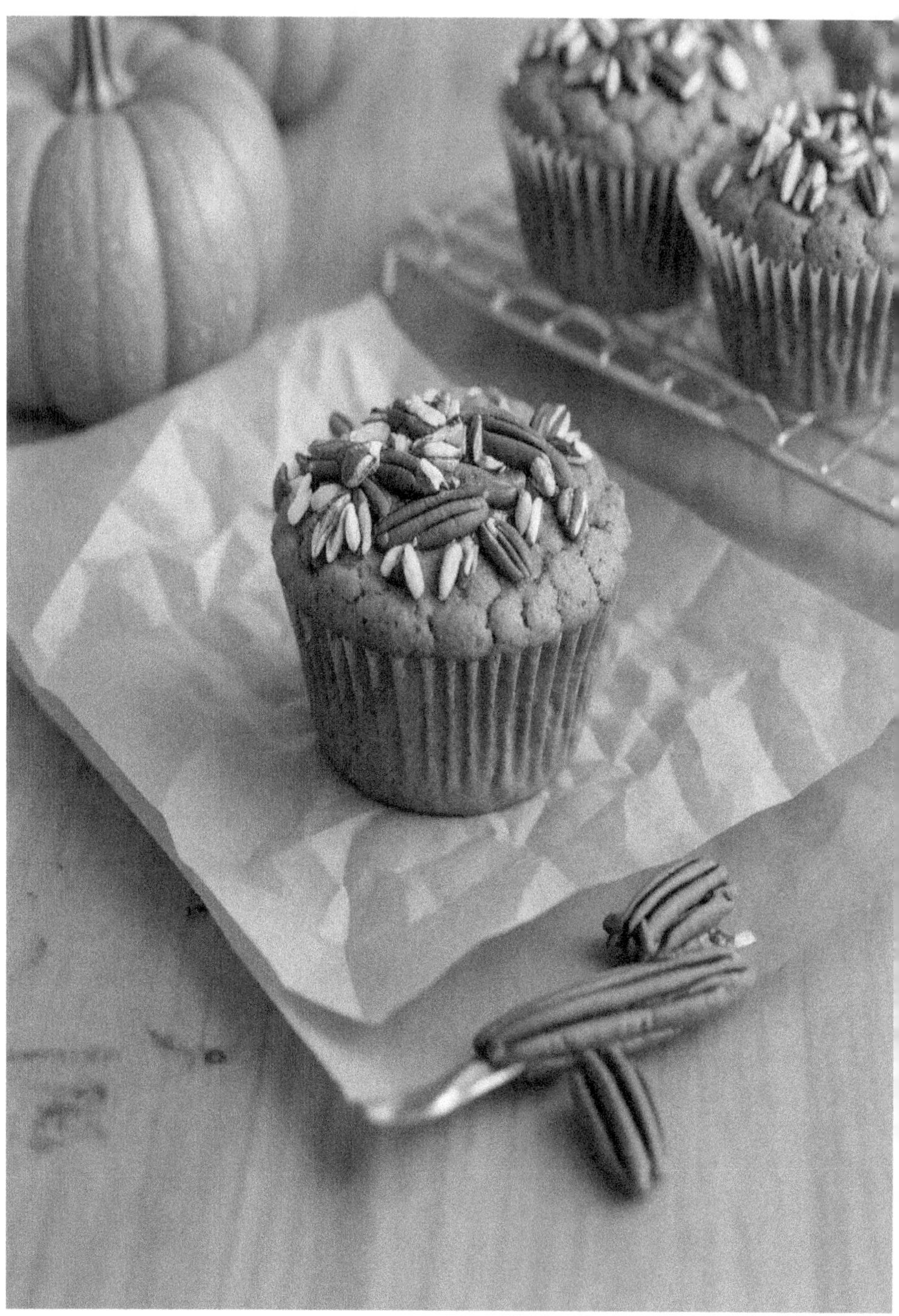

TABLE OF CONTENTS

Chapter One

Breakfast Bliss

Fuel your mornings with vibrant, delicious, and energizing plant-based breakfasts! This chapter offers a variety of options to suit your taste buds and schedule, whether you crave a quick smoothie or a leisurely sit-down meal.

1. **Sunshine Smoothie Bowl:**
   Ingredients:
   - 1 frozen banana
   - 1 cup frozen mango
   - 1/2 cup plant-based milk
   - 1/4 cup rolled oats
   - 1/4 cup Greek yogurt (dairy-free option available)
   - Toppings (fresh berries, granola, chia seeds, sliced almonds).

   Method:
   - Blend the frozen banana, mango, and plant-based milk until smooth and creamy.
   - Pour into a bowl and top with rolled oats, yogurt, and your favorite toppings.

2. **Spicy Tofu Scramble:**
   Ingredients:
   - 1 block firm tofu (crumbled)
   - 1/2 cup chopped red onion
   - 1 bell pepper diced (any color)
   - 1/2 cup chopped mushrooms
   - 1/4 teaspoon turmeric

- ➢ 1/4 teaspoon smoked paprika
- ➢ 1/8 teaspoon chili powder
- ➢ Chopped fresh cilantro
- ➢ Avocado slices
- ➢ Whole-wheat toast

Method:

- ➢ Crumble the tofu with a fork.
- ➢ Sauté the onion, bell pepper, and mushrooms in a pan with a little oil until softened.
- ➢ Add the crumbled tofu, spices, and a splash of water.
- ➢ Cook for 5-7 minutes, stirring frequently, until heated through.
- ➢ Serve on whole-wheat toast with avocado slices and fresh cilantro.

3. Power-Packed Chia Pudding:

Ingredients:

- ➢ 1/2 cup chia seeds
- ➢ 1 cup plant-based milk
- ➢ 1/4 cup chopped nuts
- ➢ 1/4 cup chopped dried fruit
- ➢ 1 teaspoon maple syrup (optional)
- ➢ 1/2 teaspoon vanilla extract

Method:

- ➢ In a jar or container, whisk together chia seeds, plant-based milk, nuts, dried fruit, maple syrup (if using) and vanilla extract.
- ➢ Cover and refrigerate overnight or for at least 4 hours. Enjoy chilled, topped with additional fruit and nuts if desired.

4. **Savory Oatmeal with Herbs and Roasted Vegetables:**
Ingredients:
  - ➢ 1/2 cup rolled oats
  - ➢ 1 cup vegetable broth
  - ➢ 1/4 cup chopped vegetables (broccoli, carrots, zucchini)
  - ➢ 1 tablespoon chopped fresh herbs (parsley, thyme)
  - ➢ Salt and pepper to taste

Method:
  - ➢ In a saucepan, combine rolled oats and vegetable broth.
  - ➢ Bring to a boil, then reduce heat and simmer for 5 minutes stirring occasionally.
  - ➢ Meanwhile, roast the chopped vegetables in a preheated oven (400°F) for 10-15 minutes until tender.
  - ➢ Stir the roasted vegetables and chopped herbs into the cooked oatmeal.
  - ➢ Season with salt and pepper to taste.

5. **Breakfast Burrito Bowl:**
Ingredients:
  - ➢ 1 cup cooked brown rice
  - ➢ 1/2 black beans (canned, drained, and rinsed)
  - ➢ 1/4 cup chopped salsa
  - ➢ 1/4 cup sliced avocado
  - ➢ 1 scrambled egg (vegan option: use a chickpea flour scramble)
  - ➢ Chopped fresh cilantro
  - ➢ Lime wedges

Method:

- ➢ Prepare brown rice according to package instructions.
- ➢ In a bowl, combine cooked brown rice, black beans, salsa, avocado, scrambled egg (or chickpea scramble), and fresh cilantro.
- ➢ Serve with lime wedges for squeezing.

6. Superfood Pancakes:

Ingredients:

- ➢ 1 ripe banana (mashed)
- ➢ 1/2 cup rolled oats
- ➢ 1/4 cup plant-based milk
- ➢ 1 tablespoon ground flaxseed (mixed with 3 tablespoons water and let sit for 5 minutes)
- ➢ 1/4 teaspoon baking powder
- ➢ 1/4 teaspoon cinnamon
- ➢ Toppings (fresh berries, chopped nuts, maple syrup)

Method:

- ➢ Mash the banana in a bowl.
- ➢ Add in the rolled oats, plant-based milk, flaxseed mixture, baking powder, and cinnamon.
- ➢ Mix well.
- ➢ Heat a lightly oiled pan over medium heat.
- ➢ Pour batter into small circles, cook for 2-3 minutes per side, or until golden brown.
- ➢ Serve pancakes with your favorite toppings.

7. Greek Yogurt Parfait with Granola and Berries:

Ingredients:

- ➢ 1 cup Greek yogurt (dairy-free option available)

> 1/2 cup granola
>
> 1 cup mixed berries

Method:

> Layer yogurt, granola, and berries in a parfait glass or bowl.
>
> Repeat layers for a visually appealing and delicious breakfast.

8. Sweet Potato Toast with Nut Butter and Sliced Banana:

Ingredients:

> 1 medium sweet potato (sliced, toasted)
>
> 2 tablespoons nut butter (almond, peanut, cashew)
>
> 1/2 banana (sliced)
>
> Pinch of cinnamon (optional)

Method:

> Toast the sweet potato slices in a toaster oven or pan until tender.
>
> Spread nut butter on the toasted sweet potato slices.
>
> Top with sliced banana and a sprinkle of cinnamon (optional).

9. Overnight Protein Oats:

Ingredients:

> 1/2 cup rolled oats
>
> 1/2 cup plant-based milk
>
> 1/4 cup Greek yogurt (dairy-free option available)
>
> 1 scoop protein powder (plant-based preferred)
>
> 1/4 cup chopped nuts
>
> 1/4 cup chopped dried fruit

Method:

> In a jar or container, combine rolled oats, plant-based milk, yogurt, protein powder, chopped nuts, and dried fruit.

> Cover and refrigerate overnight or for at least 4 hours.

> Enjoy chilled in the morning.

10. Breakfast Quesadilla with Black Beans and Scrambled Eggs:

Ingredients:

> 1 whole wheat tortilla

> 1/4 cup cooked black beans (canned, drained, and rinsed)

> 1 scrambled egg (vegan option: use a chickpea flour scramble)

> 1/4 cup shredded cheese (vegan option available)

> Salsa and avocado slices (optional).

Method:

> Heat a skillet over medium heat.

> Spread half of the shredded cheese on one half of the tortilla.

> Top with black beans and scrambled egg (or chickpea scramble).

> Fold the tortilla in half and cook for 2-3 minutes per side, or until cheese is melted and tortilla is golden brown.

> Serve with salsa and avocado slices (optional).

11. Morning Glory Muffins:

Ingredients:

> 1 ½ cups rolled oats

> 1/2 cup chopped walnuts

> 1/4 cup ground flaxseed

> 1 teaspoon baking powder

> 1/2 teaspoon cinnamon

> 1 cup mashed banana

> 1/2 cup plant-based milk

> 1/4 cup chopped dried fruit (raisins, cranberries)

> 1/4 cup chopped pitted dates.

Method:

- ➢ Preheat oven to 375°F (190°C).
- ➢ In a large bowl, combine rolled oats, walnuts, flaxseed, baking powder, and cinnamon.
- ➢ In a separate bowl, whisk together mashed banana, plant-based milk, and chopped fruit.
- ➢ Add the wet ingredients to the dry ingredients and mix until just combined.
- ➢ Fold in chopped dates. Spoon batter into greased muffin tins.
- ➢ Bake for 20-25 minutes, or until a toothpick inserted into the center comes out clean.

12. French Toast with Berries and Chia Seed Syrup:

Ingredients:

- ➢ 2 slices whole-wheat bread
- ➢ 1/2 cup plant-based milk
- ➢ 1/4 cup unsweetened applesauce
- ➢ 1 tablespoon ground flaxseed (mixed with 3 tablespoons water and let sit for 5 minutes)
- ➢ 1/4 teaspoon vanilla extract
- ➢ 1/4 teaspoon cinnamon
- ➢ 1 cup mixed berries
- ➢ maple syrup (optional).

Method:

- ➢ In a shallow bowl, whisk together plant-based milk, applesauce, flaxseed mixture, vanilla extract, and cinnamon.

- Dip each bread slice into the batter, coating both sides.
- Heat a lightly oiled pan over medium heat.
- Cook the french toast for 2-3 minutes per side, or until golden brown.
- Serve with fresh berries and a drizzle of maple syrup (optional).

13. Tofu Scramble with Turmeric and Greens:

Ingredients:

- 1 block firm tofu (crumbled)
- 1/2 cup chopped spinach or kale
- 1/4 cup chopped red onion
- 1 clove garlic (minced)
- 1/2 teaspoon turmeric
- 1/4 teaspoon smoked paprika
- Salt and pepper to taste
- Chopped fresh herbs (optional).

Method:

- Crumble the tofu with a fork.
- Sauté the red onion and garlic in a pan with a little oil until softened.
- Add the crumbled tofu, turmeric, paprika, and spinach or kale.
- Cook for 5-7 minutes, stirring frequently, until heated through.
- Season with salt and pepper to taste.
- Garnish with fresh herbs (optional) and serve with whole-wheat toast.

14. Hearty Breakfast Bowl with Quinoa and Roasted Vegetables:

Ingredients:

- ➢ 1/2 cup cooked quinoa
- ➢ 1/2 cup roasted vegetables (sweet potato, broccoli, bell peppers)
- ➢ 1/4 cup chopped avocado
- ➢ 1/4 cup black beans (canned, drained, and rinsed)
- ➢ Salsa
- ➢ Chopped fresh cilantro
- ➢ Lime wedges

Method:

- ➢ Prepare quinoa according to package instructions.
- ➢ Roast your favorite vegetables in a preheated oven (400°F) for 10-15 minutes until tender.
- ➢ In a bowl, combine cooked quinoa, roasted vegetables, avocado, black beans, salsa, and chopped cilantro.
- ➢ Serve with lime wedges for squeezing.

15. Baked Oatmeal with Apples and Walnuts:

Ingredients:

- ➢ 1 cup rolled oats
- ➢ 1 cup plant-based milk
- ➢ 1/2 cup unsweetened applesauce
- ➢ 1/4 cup chopped walnuts
- ➢ 1/4 cup chopped apple
- ➢ 1 tablespoon ground flaxseed (mixed with 3 tablespoons water and let sit for 5 minutes)
- ➢ 1/4 teaspoon baking powder
- ➢ 1/4 teaspoon cinnamon
- ➢ 1/4 teaspoon nutmeg
- ➢ Pinch of salt

Method:

- ➢ Preheat oven to 375°F (190°C).

> In a bowl, combine rolled oats, plant-based milk, applesauce, flaxseed mixture, baking powder, cinnamon, nutmeg, and salt.
> Fold in chopped walnuts and apples.
> Pour batter into a greased baking dish.
> Bake for 25-30 minutes, or until golden brown and set.

16. Chia Seed Pudding with Mango and Coconut Flakes:

Ingredients:

> 1/2 cup chia seeds
> 1 cup plant-based milk (coconut milk recommended)
> 1/2 cup chopped fresh mango
> 1/4 cup unsweetened shredded coconut
> 1 tablespoon maple syrup (optional)

Method:

> In a jar or container, whisk together chia seeds, plant-based milk, and maple syrup (if using).
> Stir in chopped mango.
> Cover and refrigerate overnight or for at least 4 hours.
> Enjoy chilled in the morning, topped with shredded coconut.

17. Hempseed and Berry Smoothie:

Ingredients:

> 1 frozen banana
> 1 cup frozen berries (mixed or your favorite kind)
> 1/2 cup plant-based milk
> 1/4 cup chopped spinach
> 2 tablespoons hemp seeds
> 1 tablespoon chia seeds
> 1 teaspoon vanilla extract

Method:

> ➢ Blend all ingredients together in a high-powered blender until smooth and creamy.
> ➢ Enjoy immediately for a refreshing and energizing breakfast.

18. Breakfast Tacos with Scrambled Eggs and Black Beans:

Ingredients:

> ➢ 2 corn tortillas
> ➢ 1 scrambled egg (vegan option: use a chickpea flour scramble)
> ➢ 1/4 cup cooked black beans (canned, drained, and rinsed)
> ➢ Salsa
> ➢ Chopped avocado
> ➢ Chopped fresh cilantro.

Method:

> ➢ Heat corn tortillas in a dry skillet or pan over medium heat for a few seconds until warmed through.
> ➢ Scramble an egg or prepare chickpea flour scramble.
> ➢ Fill each tortilla with scrambled egg, black beans, salsa, avocado, and cilantro.

19. High-Protein Pancakes with Chia Seeds and Berries:

Ingredients:

> ➢ 1 ripe banana (mashed)
> ➢ 1/2 cup rolled oats
> ➢ 1/4 cup plant-based milk
> ➢ 1 scoop protein powder (plant-based preferred)
> ➢ 1 tablespoon chia seeds
> ➢ 1/4 teaspoon baking powder
> ➢ 1/4 teaspoon cinnamon

> ➢ 1/4 cup mixed berries

Method:
- ➢ Mash the banana in a bowl.
- ➢ Add in the rolled oats, plant-based milk, protein powder, chia seeds, baking powder, and cinnamon.
- ➢ Mix well.
- ➢ Fold in half of the mixed berries.
- ➢ Heat a lightly oiled pan over medium heat.
- ➢ Pour batter into small circles, cook for 2-3 minutes per side, or until golden brown.
- ➢ Top pancakes with remaining berries and enjoy.

20. Spiced Pumpkin Muffins with Pecans:

Ingredients:
- ➢ 1 ½ cups whole wheat flour
- ➢ 1 teaspoon baking powder
- ➢ 1/2 teaspoon baking soda
- ➢ 1/2 teaspoon cinnamon
- ➢ 1/4 teaspoon nutmeg
- ➢ 1/4 teaspoon ginger
- ➢ 1 cup canned pumpkin puree
- ➢ 1/2 cup plant-based milk
- ➢ 1/4 cup maple syrup
- ➢ 1/4 cup chopped pecans
- ➢ 1/4 cup chopped dried cranberries (optional).

Method:
- ➢ Preheat oven to 375°F (190°C).
- ➢ In a large bowl, whisk together flour, baking powder, baking soda, spices.
- ➢ In a separate bowl, whisk together pumpkin puree, plant-based milk, and maple syrup.

- ➤ Add the wet ingredients to the dry ingredients and mix until just combined.
- ➤ Fold in chopped pecans and dried cranberries (if using).
- ➤ Spoon batter into greased muffin tins.
- ➤ Bake for 20-25 minutes, or until a toothpick inserted into the center comes out clean.

Tips:

- Prepare breakfast ingredients in advance, such as chopping vegetables or cooking brown rice, to save time in the mornings.
- Double or triple recipes to have leftovers for quick grab-and-go breakfasts throughout the week.
- Experiment with different plant-based milks, nuts, seeds, and fruits to personalize these recipes.
- Get creative with toppings! Fresh herbs, nutritional yeast, and a drizzle of maple syrup can add extra flavor and nutrients.

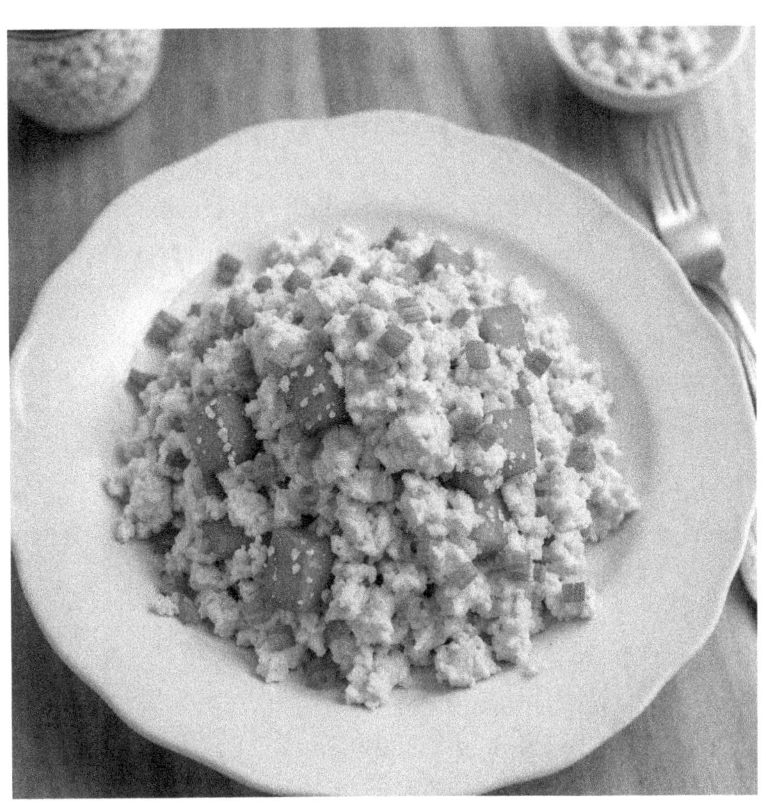

Chapter Two
Lunchtime Powerhouses

Conquer your midday cravings with these satisfying and delicious plant-based lunch options! This chapter offers a variety of recipes designed to be quick and easy to prepare, perfect for busy schedules. Whether you crave a light salad, a hearty soup, a protein-packed wrap, or a flavorful grain bowl, you'll find something to fuel your afternoon and keep you energized.

1. **Rainbow Veggie Wrap with Hummus and Sprouts:**
   Ingredients:
   - 1 whole wheat tortilla
   - 1/4 cup hummus
   - 1/4 cup chopped lettuce
   - 1/4 cup shredded carrots
   - 1/4 cup chopped cucumber
   - 1/4 cup sliced bell peppers (any color)
   - 1/4 cup alfalfa sprouts.

   Method:
   - Spread hummus evenly on a whole wheat tortilla.
   - Layer with chopped lettuce, shredded carrots, chopped cucumber, sliced bell peppers, and alfalfa sprouts.
   - Roll up tightly and enjoy!

2. **Lentil Soup with Whole Wheat Bread:**
   Ingredients:
   - 1 cup brown lentils (rinsed)
   - 4 cups vegetable broth
   - 1 cup chopped vegetables (carrots, celery, onion)
   - 2 cloves garlic (minced)

- ➢ 1 teaspoon dried thyme
- ➢ 1/2 teaspoon ground cumin
- ➢ Salt and pepper to taste
- ➢ Whole wheat bread for serving

Method:

- ➢ In a large pot, combine lentils, vegetable broth, chopped vegetables, garlic, thyme, and cumin.
- ➢ Bring to a boil, then reduce heat and simmer for 30-35 minutes, or until lentils are tender.
- ➢ Season with salt and pepper to taste.
- ➢ Serve hot with a slice of whole wheat bread.

3. **Quinoa Salad with Edamame and Tahini Dressing:**

Ingredients:

- ➢ 1 cup cooked quinoa
- ➢ 1/2 cup shelled edamame (frozen or fresh)
- ➢ 1/4 cup chopped cucumber
- ➢ 1/4 cup chopped red onion
- ➢ 1/4 cup chopped cherry tomatoes
- ➢ 1/4 cup chopped fresh parsley.

For the Tahini Dressing:

- ➢ 2 tablespoons tahini paste
- ➢ 2 tablespoons lemon juice
- ➢ 1 tablespoon olive oil
- ➢ 1 clove garlic, minced
- ➢ 1/4 cup water
- ➢ Pinch of salt
- ➢ Pinch of black pepper

Method:

- ➢ In a large bowl, combine cooked quinoa, edamame, cucumber, red onion, cherry tomatoes, and fresh parsley.

Dressing Method:

- ➢ In a separate bowl, whisk together tahini paste, lemon juice, olive oil, garlic, water, salt, and pepper.
- ➢ Pour dressing over the quinoa salad and toss to coat.

4. **Black Bean Burgers with Sweet Potato Fries:**

Ingredients (for Burgers):

- ➢ 1 can (15 oz) black beans (drained and rinsed)
- ➢ 1/2 cup cooked brown rice
- ➢ 1/4 cup chopped red onion
- ➢ 1/4 cup chopped bell pepper (any color)
- ➢ 1/4 cup chopped breadcrumbs
- ➢ 2 tablespoons chopped fresh cilantro
- ➢ 1 tablespoon olive oil
- ➢ 1 teaspoon ground cumin
- ➢ 1/2 teaspoon chili powder
- ➢ Salt and pepper to taste

Ingredients (for Sweet Potato Fries):

- ➢ 1 medium sweet potato, cut into wedges
- ➢ 1 tablespoon olive oil
- ➢ 1/2 teaspoon paprika
- ➢ 1/4 teaspoon garlic powder
- ➢ Salt and pepper to taste

Method (for Burgers):

- ➢ In a large bowl, mash together black beans with a fork (leave some texture).
- ➢ Add cooked brown rice, red onion, bell pepper, breadcrumbs, cilantro, olive oil, cumin, chili powder, salt, and pepper.
- ➢ Mix well to combine.
- ➢ Form the mixture into 4 patties.

Method (for Sweet Potato Fries):

➢ Preheat oven to 400°F (200°C).

➢ Toss sweet potato wedges with olive oil, paprika, garlic powder, salt, and pepper.

➢ Spread on a baking sheet and bake for 20-25 minutes, or until tender and lightly browned, flipping halfway through cooking.

Final Assembly:

➢ Heat a lightly oiled pan over medium heat.

➢ Cook black bean burgers for 3-4 minutes per side, or until heated through.

➢ Serve burgers on hamburger buns with your favorite toppings and a side of sweet potato fries.

5. **Creamy Tomato Pasta with Chickpeas and Spinach:**

Ingredients:

➢ 1 pound whole wheat pasta (penne, rotini, or your favorite shape)

➢ 1 (14.5 oz) can diced tomatoes, undrained

➢ 1 cup cooked chickpeas (canned, drained, and rinsed)

➢ 1/2 cup chopped red onion

➢ 2 cloves garlic (minced)

➢ 1/2 cup vegetable broth

➢ 1/4 cup vegan cream cheese (or dairy-free alternative)

➢ 1/4 cup chopped fresh basil

➢ 1 tablespoon olive oil

➢ 1 teaspoon dried oregano

➢ Salt and pepper to taste

Method:

➢ Cook whole wheat pasta according to package instructions.

➢ Meanwhile, heat olive oil in a large pan over medium heat.

- ➢ Add red onion and garlic, cook for 2-3 minutes, or until softened.
- ➢ Stir in diced tomatoes, vegetable broth, oregano, salt, and pepper.
- ➢ Bring to a simmer and cook for 5 minutes.
- ➢ Add cooked chickpeas and vegan cream cheese.
- ➢ Stir until cream cheese is melted and sauce is creamy.
- ➢ Drain cooked pasta and add it to the pan with the tomato sauce.
- ➢ Toss to coat.
- ➢ Stir in chopped fresh basil and serve immediately.

6. **Mediterranean Chickpea Salad Sandwich on Whole Wheat Bread:**

Ingredients:
- ➢ 1 can (15 oz) chickpeas, drained and rinsed
- ➢ 1/2 cup chopped cucumber
- ➢ 1/4 cup chopped red onion
- ➢ 1/4 cup chopped cherry tomatoes
- ➢ 1/4 cup crumbled feta cheese (vegan option available)
- ➢ 2 tablespoons chopped Kalamata olives
- ➢ 2 tablespoons olive oil
- ➢ 1 tablespoon lemon juice
- ➢ 1/2 teaspoon dried oregano
- ➢ Salt and pepper to taste
- ➢ 2 slices whole wheat bread

Method:
- ➢ In a large bowl, combine chickpeas, cucumber, red onion, cherry tomatoes, feta cheese (or vegan alternative), and Kalamata olives.

- In a separate bowl, whisk together olive oil, lemon juice, oregano, salt, and pepper.
- Pour dressing over the chickpea mixture and toss to coat.
- Toast whole wheat bread slices (optional).
- Spread chickpea salad on toasted bread slices and enjoy!

7. Spicy Edamame and Veggie Bowl with Brown Rice:

Ingredients:

- 1 cup cooked brown rice
- 1 cup steamed or roasted vegetables (broccoli, carrots, zucchini)
- 1/2 cup shelled edamame (frozen or fresh)
- 1/4 cup sliced avocado
- 1/4 cup chopped fresh cilantro
- 1 tablespoon sesame seeds

For the Spicy Peanut Sauce:

- 2 tablespoons peanut butter
- 2 tablespoons soy sauce (or tamari for gluten-free)
- 1 tablespoon rice vinegar
- 1 tablespoon sriracha (or less for a milder sauce)
- 1 tablespoon water
- 1 clove garlic, minced

Method:

- Prepare brown rice according to package instructions. Steam or roast vegetables until tender-crisp.
- Cook edamame according to package instructions (if using frozen).

Dressing Method:

- In a small bowl, whisk together peanut butter, soy sauce, rice vinegar, sriracha, water, and garlic.

Final Assembly:

> ➤ In a bowl, combine cooked brown rice, roasted vegetables, edamame, sliced avocado, and chopped cilantro.
> ➤ Drizzle with spicy peanut sauce and sprinkle with sesame seeds.

8. **Rainbow Veggie Wrap with Hummus and Quinoa:**
Ingredients:

> ➤ 1 large whole wheat tortilla
> ➤ 1/2 cup cooked quinoa
> ➤ 1/4 cup hummus
> ➤ 1/4 cup shredded carrots
> ➤ 1/4 cup chopped cucumber
> ➤ 1/4 cup chopped bell peppers (any color)
> ➤ 1/4 cup chopped spinach or kale

Method:

> ➤ Spread hummus evenly on a whole wheat tortilla. Layer with cooked quinoa, shredded carrots, chopped cucumber, bell peppers, and spinach or kale. Roll up tightly and enjoy!

9. **Curried Chickpea Salad Pita Pockets:**
Ingredients:

> ➤ 1 can (15 oz) chickpeas, drained and rinsed
> ➤ 1/2 cup chopped celery
> ➤ 1/4 cup chopped red onion
> ➤ 1/4 cup chopped cucumber
> ➤ 1/4 cup chopped red onion
> ➤ 1/4 cup chopped cucumber
> ➤ 1/4 cup chopped fresh cilantro
> ➤ 2 tablespoons raisins (optional)
> ➤ 2 tablespoons chopped walnuts (optional)

- ➢ 2 tablespoons curry powder
- ➢ 1 tablespoon olive oil
- ➢ 1 tablespoon lemon juice
- ➢ 1/2 teaspoon ground cumin
- ➢ Salt and pepper to taste
- ➢ 2 whole wheat pita breads

Method:

- ➢ In a large bowl, combine chickpeas, celery, red onion, cucumber, cilantro, raisins (if using), and walnuts (if using).
- ➢ In a separate bowl, whisk together curry powder, olive oil, lemon juice, cumin, salt, and pepper.
- ➢ Pour dressing over the chickpea mixture and toss to coat.
- ➢ Warm whole wheat pita breads according to package instructions (microwave or toaster oven).
- ➢ Stuff pita breads with curried chickpea salad and enjoy!

10. Asian Noodle Salad with Peanut Dressing:

Ingredients:

- ➢ 8 ounces brown rice noodles or rice noodles of choice
- ➢ 1 cup chopped vegetables (shredded carrots, bean sprouts, julienned red bell pepper)
- ➢ 1/2 cup chopped cucumber
- ➢ 1/4 cup chopped fresh cilantro
- ➢ 1/4 cup chopped roasted peanuts

For the Peanut Dressing:

- ➢ 2 tablespoons peanut butter
- ➢ 2 tablespoons soy sauce (or tamari for gluten-free)
- ➢ 1 tablespoon rice vinegar
- ➢ 1 tablespoon sesame oil
- ➢ 1 tablespoon lime juice

- ➢ 1 clove garlic, minced
- ➢ 1 teaspoon grated ginger

Method:

- ➢ Cook brown rice noodles according to package instructions. Drain and rinse with cold water.
- ➢ In a large bowl, combine cooked noodles, chopped vegetables, cilantro, and roasted peanuts.

Dressing Method:

- ➢ In a small bowl, whisk together peanut butter, soy sauce, rice vinegar, sesame oil, lime juice, garlic, and ginger.

Final Assembly:

- ➢ Pour peanut dressing over the noodle and vegetable mixture and toss to coat.
- ➢ Serve immediately.

11. Veggie Burger on a Kaiser Roll with Avocado Mayo:

Ingredients (for Veggie Burger):

- ➢ 1 cup cooked brown rice
- ➢ 1/2 cup mashed black beans
- ➢ 1/4 cup chopped mushrooms
- ➢ 1/4 cup chopped red onion
- ➢ 1/4 cup breadcrumbs
- ➢ 2 tablespoons chopped fresh parsley
- ➢ 1 tablespoon olive oil
- ➢ 1 teaspoon ground cumin
- ➢ 1/2 teaspoon smoked paprika
- ➢ Salt and pepper to taste

Ingredients (for Avocado Mayo):

- ➢ 1/2 ripe avocado, mashed
- ➢ 2 tablespoons vegan mayonnaise
- ➢ 1 tablespoon lemon juice

> ➤ Salt and pepper to taste

Other Ingredients:
- ➤ 1 kaiser roll
- ➤ Lettuce, tomato, and red onion slices (for garnish)

Method (for Veggie Burger):
- ➤ In a large bowl, combine cooked brown rice, mashed black beans, mushrooms, red onion, breadcrumbs, parsley, olive oil, cumin, smoked paprika, salt, and pepper.
- ➤ Mix well to combine.
- ➤ Form the mixture into 1 burger patty.

Method (for Avocado Mayo):
- ➤ Mash avocado in a bowl. Stir in vegan mayonnaise, lemon juice, salt, and pepper.

Final Assembly:
- ➤ Heat a lightly oiled pan over medium heat. Cook the veggie burger for 3-4 minutes per side, or until heated through.
- ➤ Toast the kaiser roll (optional).
- ➤ Spread avocado mayo on the bottom half of the roll.
- ➤ Top with lettuce, tomato, red onion slices, and the veggie burger. Enjoy!

12. Thai Coconut Curry Soup with Vegetables and Tofu:

Ingredients:
- ➤ 1 tablespoon olive oil
- ➤ 1 onion (chopped)
- ➤ 2 cloves garlic (minced)
- ➤ 1 tablespoon curry powder
- ➤ 1 teaspoon ground ginger
- ➤ 1 (13.5 oz) can coconut milk
- ➤ 4 cups vegetable broth
- ➤ 1 cup chopped vegetables (broccoli, carrots, bell peppers)

> ➢ 1 block firm tofu, drained and cubed
> ➢ 1 cup cooked brown rice (optional)
> ➢ Fresh cilantro, chopped (for garnish)
> ➢ Lime wedges (for garnish)

Method:

> ➢ Heat olive oil in a large pot over medium heat.
> ➢ Add onion and garlic, cook for 2-3 minutes, or until softened.
> ➢ Stir in curry powder and ginger, cook for an additional minute.
> ➢ Pour in coconut milk and vegetable broth. Bring to a simmer.
> ➢ Add chopped vegetables and tofu.
> ➢ Simmer for 15-20 minutes, or until vegetables are tender.
> ➢ Serve hot with cooked brown rice (optional), garnished with chopped fresh cilantro and lime wedges.

13. Mediterranean Quinoa Salad with Sun-dried Tomatoes and Kalamata Olives:

Ingredients:

> ➢ 1 cup cooked quinoa
> ➢ 1/2 cup chopped cucumber
> ➢ 1/4 cup chopped red onion
> ➢ 1/4 cup chopped bell peppers (any color)
> ➢ 1/4 cup crumbled feta cheese (vegan option available)
> ➢ 1/4 cup chopped sun-dried tomatoes (not packed in oil)
> ➢ 1/4 cup pitted Kalamata olives, halved
> ➢ 2 tablespoons olive oil
> ➢ 1 tablespoon lemon juice
> ➢ 1/2 teaspoon dried oregano
> ➢ Salt and pepper to taste

Method:
- In a large bowl, combine cooked quinoa, chopped cucumber, red onion, bell peppers, feta cheese (or vegan alternative), sun-dried tomatoes, and Kalamata olives.
- In a separate bowl, whisk together olive oil, lemon juice, oregano, salt, and pepper.
- Pour dressing over the quinoa salad and toss to coat.
- Serve immediately.

14. Edamame and Veggie Power Bowl with Miso Tahini Dressing:

Ingredients:
- 1 cup cooked brown rice
- 1 cup steamed or roasted vegetables (broccoli, sweet potato, Brussels sprouts)
- 1/2 cup shelled edamame (frozen or fresh)
- 1/4 cup sliced avocado
- 1/4 cup chopped fresh cilantro
- 1 tablespoon sesame seeds

For the Miso Tahini Dressing:
- 2 tablespoons white miso paste
- 2 tablespoons tahini paste
- 2 tablespoons rice vinegar
- 1 tablespoon soy sauce (or tamari for gluten-free)
- 1 tablespoon water
- 1 clove garlic, minced
- 1 teaspoon grated ginger

Method:
- Prepare brown rice according to package instructions. Steam or roast vegetables until tender-crisp.

> Cook edamame according to package instructions (if using frozen).

Dressing Method:

> In a small bowl, whisk together miso paste, tahini paste, rice vinegar, soy sauce, water, garlic, and ginger.

Final Assembly:

> In a bowl, combine cooked brown rice, roasted vegetables, edamame, sliced avocado, and chopped cilantro.

> Drizzle with miso tahini dressing and sprinkle with sesame seeds.

15. Spicy Peanut Buddha Bowl with Tofu Scramble:

Ingredients:

> 1 cup cooked quinoa
> 1/2 block firm tofu, crumbled
> 1/2 cup chopped vegetables (red onion, bell peppers)
> 1/4 cup shredded carrots
> 1/4 cup chopped fresh spinach
> 1 tablespoon olive oil
> 1/2 teaspoon turmeric
> 1/4 teaspoon smoked paprika
> Pinch of chili powder
> Salt and pepper to taste

For the Spicy Peanut Sauce:

> 2 tablespoons peanut butter
> 2 tablespoons soy sauce (or tamari for gluten-free)
> 1 tablespoon rice vinegar
> 1 tablespoon sriracha (or less for a milder sauce)
> 1 tablespoon water
> 1 clove garlic, minced

Method (for Tofu Scramble):

- ➢ Crumble the tofu with a fork.
- ➢ Heat olive oil in a pan over medium heat.
- ➢ Add crumbled tofu and cook for 5-7 minutes, stirring frequently, until golden brown.
- ➢ Season with turmeric, smoked paprika, chili powder, salt, and pepper.

Dressing Method:

- ➢ In a small bowl, whisk together peanut butter, soy sauce, rice vinegar, sriracha, water, and garlic.

Final Assembly:

- ➢ In a bowl, combine cooked quinoa, tofu scramble, chopped vegetables, shredded carrots, and fresh spinach.
- ➢ Drizzle with spicy peanut sauce and enjoy.

16. Black Bean and Corn Quesadillas with Avocado Crema:

Ingredients:

- ➢ 2 whole wheat tortillas
- ➢ 1/2 cup canned black beans, drained and rinsed
- ➢ 1/2 cup frozen corn, thawed
- ➢ 1/4 cup shredded vegan cheese (optional)
- ➢ 1/4 cup chopped red onion
- ➢ 1 tablespoon olive oil
- ➢ 1/2 teaspoon chili powder
- ➢ 1/4 teaspoon cumin
- ➢ Salt and pepper to taste

For the Avocado Crema:

- ➢ 1/2 ripe avocado, mashed
- ➢ 1 tablespoon lime juice
- ➢ 1/4 cup unsweetened plant-based yogurt (optional)
- ➢ Salt and pepper to taste

Method:

- ➢ In a pan, heat olive oil over medium heat.
- ➢ Add black beans, corn, red onion, chili powder, and cumin.
- ➢ Cook for 5-7 minutes, or until heated through.
- ➢ Season with salt and pepper.

Crema Method:

- ➢ Mash avocado in a bowl. Stir in lime juice, plant-based yogurt (if using), salt, and pepper.

Final Assembly:

- ➢ Place one tortilla on a flat surface. Spread half of the black bean and corn mixture on one half of the tortilla.
- ➢ Top with vegan cheese (if using).
- ➢ Fold the tortilla in half.
- ➢ Repeat with the second tortilla.
- ➢ Heat a lightly oiled pan or griddle over medium heat.
- ➢ Cook the quesadillas for 2-3 minutes per side, or until golden brown and crispy.
- ➢ Serve quesadillas with avocado crema for dipping.

17. Lentil Shepherd's Pie with Mashed Potatoes:

Ingredients (for Shepherd's Pie):

- ➢ 1 tablespoon olive oil
- ➢ 1 onion, chopped
- ➢ 2 cloves garlic, minced
- ➢ 1 cup cooked brown lentils
- ➢ 1 cup chopped vegetables (carrots, celery, peas)
- ➢ 1 (14.5 oz) can diced tomatoes, undrained
- ➢ 1 cup vegetable broth
- ➢ 1 tablespoon tomato paste
- ➢ 1 tablespoon Worcestershire sauce (vegan option available)
- ➢ 1 teaspoon dried thyme
- ➢ Salt and pepper to taste

Ingredients (for Mashed Potatoes):
- 2 medium potatoes, peeled and diced
- 1/4 cup plant-based milk (or unsweetened almond milk)
- 2 tablespoons vegan butter
- Salt and pepper to taste

Method (for Shepherd's Pie):
- Heat olive oil in a large pot or Dutch oven over medium heat.
- Add onion and garlic, cook for 2-3 minutes, or until softened.
- Stir in cooked brown lentils, chopped vegetables, diced tomatoes, vegetable broth, tomato paste, Worcestershire sauce, and thyme.
- Bring to a simmer and cook for 15-20 minutes, or until vegetables are tender.
- Season with salt and pepper to taste.

Method (for Mashed Potatoes):
- In a pot, cover diced potatoes with water and bring to a boil.
- Reduce heat and simmer for 15-20 minutes, or until potatoes are fork-tender.
- Drain potatoes and return them to the pot.
- Using a potato masher or hand mixer, mash potatoes until smooth.
- Add plant-based milk and vegan butter.
- Season with salt and pepper to taste.

Final Assembly:
- Preheat oven to 375°F (190°C). Preheat a baking dish while the shepherd's pie filling simmers.
- Spoon the lentil mixture into the prepared baking dish.
- Top with mashed potatoes, spreading evenly.

- ➤ Bake for 20-25 minutes, or until the edges are golden brown and bubbly.
- ➤ Let cool slightly before serving.

18. Rainbow Veggie Wrap with Hummus and Quinoa (Variation):
Ingredients:
- ➤ 1 large whole wheat tortilla
- ➤ 1/2 cup cooked quinoa
- ➤ 1/4 cup hummus
- ➤ 1/4 cup shredded carrots
- ➤ 1/4 cup chopped cucumber
- ➤ 1/4 cup chopped bell peppers (any color)
- ➤ 1/4 cup sliced avocado
- ➤ 1/4 cup chopped fresh spinach

Method:
- ➤ Spread hummus evenly on a whole wheat tortilla.
- ➤ Layer with cooked quinoa, shredded carrots, chopped cucumber, bell peppers, sliced avocado, and fresh spinach. Roll up tightly and enjoy!

19. Tofu Banh Mi Sandwich on a French Baguette:
Ingredients:
- ➤ 1 French baguette, cut in half
- ➤ 1/2 block firm tofu, marinated and pan-fried (optional marinade: soy sauce, rice vinegar, garlic, ginger)
- ➤ 1/4 cup pickled vegetables (carrots, daikon radish)
- ➤ 1/4 cup chopped cucumber
- ➤ 1/4 cup fresh cilantro
- ➤ 1 tablespoon vegan mayonnaise (or sriracha mayo)
- ➤ Sriracha sauce (optional)

Method:

- ➢ Marinate tofu according to your preferred recipe (optional).
- ➢ Pan-fry tofu slices until golden brown on both sides.
- ➢ Toast the French baguette halves (optional).
- ➢ Spread vegan mayonnaise (or sriracha mayo) on both halves of the baguette.
- ➢ Layer with tofu slices, pickled vegetables, chopped cucumber, and fresh cilantro.
- ➢ Drizzle with sriracha sauce (optional) and enjoy!

20. Hearty Chickpea and Vegetable Soup with Whole Wheat Bread:

Ingredients:

- ➢ 1 tablespoon olive oil
- ➢ 1 onion, chopped
- ➢ 2 cloves garlic, minced
- ➢ 1 (15 oz) can chickpeas, drained and rinsed
- ➢ 4 cups vegetable broth
- ➢ 2 cups chopped vegetables (carrots, celery, potatoes)
- ➢ 1 (14.5 oz) can diced tomatoes, undrained
- ➢ 1 tablespoon dried oregano
- ➢ 1 teaspoon ground cumin
- ➢ Salt and pepper to taste
- ➢ Whole wheat bread for serving

Method:

- ➢ Heat olive oil in a large pot over medium heat.
- ➢ Add onion and garlic, cook for 2-3 minutes, or until softened.
- ➢ Stir in chickpeas, vegetable broth, chopped vegetables, diced tomatoes, oregano, and cumin.
- ➢ Bring to a simmer and cook for 20-25 minutes, or until vegetables are tender. Season with salt and pepper to taste.

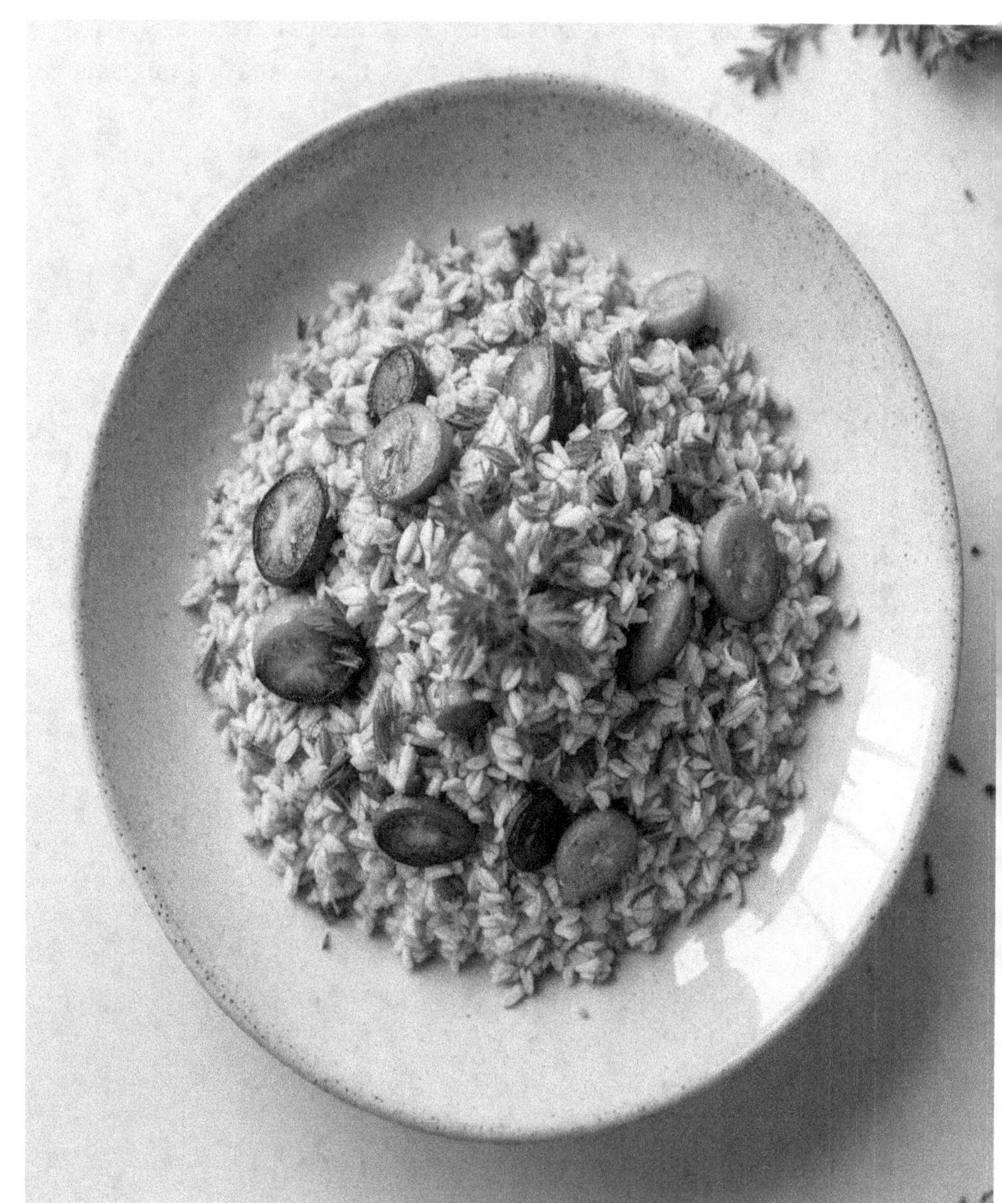

Chapter Three
Dinnertime Delights

Looking to create a showstopping plant-based meal that's both delicious and nutritious? Look no further! This chapter dives into ten impressive main courses featuring legumes, whole grains, and seasonal vegetables, guaranteed to tantalize taste buds and leave everyone wanting more.

1. **Stuffed Portobello Mushrooms with Lentil Walnut "Meat" (Vegan):**

This recipe transforms humble portobello mushrooms into a hearty and flavorful main course.

Ingredients:

- 4 large portobello mushrooms (stems removed)
- 1 cup cooked brown lentils
- 1/2 cup chopped walnuts
- 1/4 cup chopped red onion
- 2 cloves garlic, minced
- 1/2 cup chopped fresh parsley
- 1/4 cup breadcrumbs
- 1 tablespoon olive oil
- 1/2 teaspoon dried thyme
- 1/4 teaspoon smoked paprika
- Salt and pepper to taste

Method:

Preheat oven to 400°F (200°C). Brush the tops of the portobello mushrooms with olive oil and season with salt and pepper.

Place them gill-side down on a baking sheet and bake for 10 minutes.

Lentil Walnut "Meat" Filling:
- While the mushrooms bake, heat olive oil in a large skillet over medium heat.
- Add chopped onion and cook for 5 minutes, or until softened.
- Stir in minced garlic and cook for an additional minute, until fragrant.
- Add cooked brown lentils, chopped walnuts, chopped fresh parsley, breadcrumbs, dried thyme, and smoked paprika.
- Season with salt and pepper to taste.
- Cook for another 2-3 minutes, allowing the flavors to meld.

Assembling and Finishing:
- Remove the portobello mushrooms from the oven and carefully flip them over.
- Spoon the lentil walnut filling evenly into the portobello caps.
- Return the stuffed mushrooms to the baking sheet and bake for an additional 15-20 minutes, or until the filling is heated through and the tops are golden brown.
- Serve hot with a side of roasted vegetables or quinoa.

2. Moroccan Chickpea Tagine with Couscous (Vegan):

This aromatic tagine transports you to North Africa with its blend of spices and chickpeas.

Ingredients:
- 2 tablespoons olive oil
- 1 medium onion, chopped
- 2 cloves garlic, minced
- 1 teaspoon ground ginger
- 1/2 teaspoon ground cumin

- ➢ 1/4 teaspoon turmeric
- ➢ Pinch of saffron threads (optional)
- ➢ 1 (14.5 oz) can diced tomatoes, undrained
- ➢ 4 cups vegetable broth
- ➢ 1 (15 oz) can chickpeas, rinsed and drained
- ➢ 1 cup chopped carrots
- ➢ 1 cup chopped zucchini
- ➢ 1/2 cup chopped fresh parsley
- ➢ 1 cup cooked couscous
- ➢ Toasted almonds and chopped fresh cilantro, for garnish (optional)

Method:

Heat olive oil in a large pot or Dutch oven over medium heat.

Add chopped onion and cook for 5 minutes, or until softened.

Stir in minced garlic, ginger, cumin, turmeric, and saffron threads (if using).

Cook for an additional minute, allowing the spices to release their aroma.

Adding Liquids and Base:

- ➢ Pour in diced tomatoes with their juices and vegetable broth.
- ➢ Bring to a boil, then reduce heat and simmer for 10 minutes.
- ➢ Stir in rinsed and drained chickpeas, chopped carrots, and chopped zucchini.
- ➢ Simmer for an additional 20-25 minutes, or until the vegetables are tender-crisp.

Finishing Touches:

- ➢ Season the tagine with salt and pepper to taste.
- ➢ Stir in chopped fresh parsley.
- ➢ Serve hot over a bed of cooked couscous.

> Garnish with toasted almonds and chopped fresh cilantro (optional).

3. Lemony Quinoa Stuffed Peppers with Black Beans and Corn (Vegetarian):

This vibrant dish is a protein and fiber-packed meal perfect for a light yet satisfying dinner.

Ingredients:
- 4 large bell peppers (any color combination)
- 1 cup cooked quinoa
- 1 (15 oz) can black beans, rinsed and drained
- 1 cup frozen corn, thawed
- 1/2 cup chopped red onion
- 2 cloves garlic, minced
- 1/4 cup chopped fresh cilantro
- 1 tablespoon olive oil
- 1 tablespoon lemon juice
- 1/2 teaspoon ground cumin
- 1/4 cup crumbled feta cheese (vegan option available)
- Salt and pepper to taste

Method:
- Preheat oven to 400°F (200°C).
- Cut the tops off the bell peppers and remove the seeds and membranes.
- Rinse the peppers and place them cut-side up on a baking sheet.

Quinoa Stuffing:
- In a large bowl, combine cooked quinoa, rinsed and drained black beans, thawed corn, chopped red onion, minced garlic, chopped fresh cilantro, olive oil, lemon juice,

ground cumin, and crumbled feta cheese (or vegan alternative).
- ➢ Season with salt and pepper to taste.
- ➢ Mix well to combine.

Stuffing and Baking:
- ➢ Spoon the quinoa stuffing mixture evenly into the hollowed-out bell peppers.
- ➢ Bake the stuffed peppers for 20-25 minutes, or until the peppers are tender and the filling is heated through.

Serving Suggestion:
- ➢ Serve hot with a side salad or roasted vegetables.

4. **Ethiopian Spicy Lentil Stew (Shiro Wat) with Injera (Vegan):**

This flavorful Ethiopian stew features lentils simmered in a fragrant berbere spice blend, perfect with injera flatbread.

Ingredients (for Shiro Wat):
- ➢ 2 tablespoons vegetable oil
- ➢ 1 medium onion, chopped
- ➢ 2 cloves garlic, minced
- ➢ 1 tablespoon grated ginger
- ➢ 2 teaspoons berbere spice blend
- ➢ 1 (14.5 oz) can diced tomatoes (undrained)
- ➢ 4 cups vegetable broth
- ➢ 1 cup red lentils, rinsed and drained
- ➢ Salt and pepper to taste

Ingredients (for Injera - optional):
- ➢ 2 cups teff flour
- ➢ 3/4 cup warm water
- ➢ 1/2 teaspoon sugar
- ➢ Pinch of salt

Method (for Shiro Wat):

- ➤ Heat vegetable oil in a large pot or Dutch oven over medium heat.
- ➤ Add chopped onion and cook for 5 minutes, or until softened.
- ➤ Stir in minced garlic and grated ginger.
- ➤ Cook for an additional minute, until fragrant.
- ➤ Add berbere spice blend and cook for another minute, allowing the spices to release their aroma.

Adding Liquids and Base:

- ➤ Pour in diced tomatoes with their juices and vegetable broth.
- ➤ Bring to a boil, then reduce heat and simmer for 10 minutes.
- ➤ Stir in rinsed and drained red lentils.
- ➤ Simmer for an additional 30-35 minutes, or until the lentils are tender and the stew has thickened slightly.

Seasoning and Injera (Optional):

- ➤ Season the stew with salt and pepper to taste.

Injera (Optional):

- ➤ If making injera, combine teff flour, warm water, sugar, and salt in a large bowl.
- ➤ Whisk well until smooth and slightly bubbly. Let the batter rest for at least 2 hours, or preferably overnight, at room temperature.
- ➤ Heat a lightly oiled non-stick skillet or griddle over medium heat.
- ➤ Pour a ladleful of batter onto the skillet and swirl to form a thin crepe-like circle.
- ➤ Cook for 1-2 minutes per side, or until the edges become slightly crisp.

> Injera should be slightly fermented and have a spongy texture.

Serving Suggestion:
> Serve the Shiro Wat stew spooned onto injera flatbread (if making) or with rice or another grain of your choice.

5. Rainbow Veggie Buddha Bowl with Tahini Sauce (Vegan):

This customizable bowl allows you to showcase a variety of seasonal vegetables and roasted chickpeas for a protein punch.

Ingredients (for Tahini Sauce):
> 1/2 cup tahini
> 1/4 cup lemon juice
> 2 cloves garlic (minced)
> 2-3 tablespoons water
> Salt and pepper to taste

Ingredients (for the Bowl):
> 1 cup assorted roasted vegetables (such as broccoli, Brussels sprouts, sweet potato, carrots)
> 1 cup cooked quinoa or brown rice
> 1 can (15 oz) chickpeas, rinsed and drained
> 1/2 cup chopped cucumber
> 1/4 cup crumbled feta cheese (vegan option available)
> 1/4 cup chopped fresh herbs (such as parsley, cilantro, or mint)
> Additional toppings (optional): avocado slices, roasted nuts, seeds

Method (for Tahini Sauce):
> In a small bowl, whisk together tahini, lemon juice, minced garlic, and water until smooth and creamy.
> Season with salt.

Method (for Roasted Vegetables):

> ➤ Preheat oven to 400°F (200°C).
> ➤ Toss your chosen assorted vegetables (broccoli, Brussels sprouts, sweet potato, carrots, etc.) with olive oil, salt, and pepper.
> ➤ Spread them out on a baking sheet in a single layer and roast for 20-25 minutes, or until tender-crisp and slightly browned.

Preparing Chickpeas:

> ➤ While the vegetables roast, toss the rinsed and drained chickpeas with olive oil, a sprinkle of cumin, and chili powder (optional).
> ➤ Spread them on a separate baking sheet and roast for 15-20 minutes, or until golden brown and crispy.

Assembling the Bowl:

> ➤ Divide cooked quinoa or brown rice among serving bowls. Top with roasted vegetables, crispy chickpeas, chopped cucumber, crumbled feta cheese (or vegan alternative), and chopped fresh herbs.
> ➤ Drizzle generously with tahini sauce and garnish with additional toppings like avocado slices, roasted nuts, or seeds (optional).

6. Hearty Korean Bibimbap with Gochujang Sauce (Vegetarian Option):

This colorful Korean dish features seasoned vegetables, rice, and a fried egg, all served in a heated stone pot for a sizzling presentation.

Ingredients (for Gochujang Sauce):

> ➤ 2 tablespoons gochujang (Korean chili paste)

- ➤ 1 tablespoon soy sauce
- ➤ 1 tablespoon rice vinegar
- ➤ 1 tablespoon sesame oil
- ➤ 1 clove garlic, minced
- ➤ 1 teaspoon honey or agave nectar (optional)

Ingredients (for Bibimbap):
- ➤ 1 cup cooked white rice
- ➤ 1 cup assorted vegetables (such as julienned carrots, zucchini, spinach, bean sprouts)
- ➤ 1 portobello mushroom, sliced and marinated in soy sauce (optional)
- ➤ 1 fried egg per serving
- ➤ Sesame seeds and chopped scallions, for garnish

Method (for Gochujang Sauce):
- ➤ In a small bowl, whisk together gochujang, soy sauce, rice vinegar, sesame oil, minced garlic, and honey (if using).
- ➤ Adjust the amount of gochujang to your desired spice level.

Preparing Vegetables:
- ➤ Sauté each vegetable separately in a pan with a little oil until tender-crisp.
- ➤ You can also blanch them in boiling water for a minute and then shock them in ice water to retain their vibrant colors.

Assembling the Bibimbap:
- ➤ If using a dolsot (heated stone pot), preheat it according to package instructions.
- ➤ Alternatively, use a regular bowl.
- ➤ Divide cooked white rice among the bowls.
- ➤ Arrange the seasoned vegetables in sections around the rice, leaving a well in the center.
- ➤ Slide a fried egg into the well of each bowl.

- ➢ Drizzle generously with gochujang sauce.
- ➢ Garnish with sesame seeds and chopped scallions.

7. Thai Green Curry with Vegetables and Tofu (Vegan):

This fragrant curry showcases vibrant green vegetables simmered in a creamy coconut milk base with tofu.

Ingredients:
- ➢ 2 tablespoons vegetable oil
- ➢ 1 green bell pepper (chopped)
- ➢ 1 red bell pepper (chopped)
- ➢ 1 cup broccoli florets
- ➢ 1 cup green beans (trimmed and chopped)
- ➢ 1 (14 oz) can coconut milk
- ➢ 1 cup vegetable broth
- ➢ 1 tablespoon green curry paste
- ➢ 1 block firm tofu (drained and cubed)
- ➢ 1 tablespoon soy sauce
- ➢ 1 tablespoon lime juice
- ➢ 1 tablespoon brown sugar
- ➢ 1 cup cooked rice or noodles (for serving)
- ➢ Fresh cilantro and lime wedges, for garnish (optional)

Method:
- ➢ Heat vegetable oil in a large pot or Dutch oven over medium heat.
- ➢ Add chopped bell peppers, broccoli florets, and green beans
- ➢ Sauté for 5 minutes, or until slightly softened.

Adding Liquids and Base:

- ➢ Pour in coconut milk and vegetable broth.
- ➢ Stir in green curry paste, cubed tofu, soy sauce, lime juice, and brown sugar.
- ➢ Bring to a simmer and cook for 15-20 minutes, or until the vegetables are tender and the tofu is heated through.

Finishing Touches:
- ➢ Serve the Thai green curry hot over cooked rice or noodles.
- ➢ Garnish with fresh cilantro and lime wedges (optional).

8. Lentil Shepherd's Pie with Mashed Potatoes (Vegan):

This hearty vegan take on shepherd's pie features a savory lentil filling topped with creamy mashed potatoes.

Ingredients (for Lentil Filling):
- ➢ 2 tablespoons olive oil
- ➢ 1 medium onion (chopped)
- ➢ 2 carrots (chopped)
- ➢ 2 celery stalks (chopped)
- ➢ 2 cloves garlic (minced)
- ➢ 1 teaspoon dried thyme
- ➢ 1/2 teaspoon ground cumin
- ➢ 1 cup brown lentils (rinsed and drained)
- ➢ 4 cups vegetable broth
- ➢ 1 (14.5 oz) can diced tomatoes (undrained)
- ➢ 1 cup frozen peas
- ➢ Salt and pepper to taste

Ingredients (for Mashed Potatoes):
- ➢ 4-5 russet potatoes, peeled and cut into cubes
- ➢ 1/2 cup vegan butter or olive oil
- ➢ 1/2 cup plant-based milk (such as soy milk or almond milk)

- ➢ Salt and pepper to taste

Method (for Lentil Filling):
- ➢ Heat olive oil in a large pot or Dutch oven over medium heat.
- ➢ Add chopped onion, carrots, and celery.
- ➢ Sauté for 5-7 minutes, or until softened.
- ➢ Stir in minced garlic, dried thyme, and ground cumin.
- ➢ Cook for an additional minute, allowing the spices to release their aroma.

Adding Broth, Vegetables, and Lentils:
- ➢ Pour in vegetable broth and diced tomatoes with their juices.
- ➢ Bring to a boil, then reduce heat and simmer for 15 minutes.
- ➢ Stir in rinsed and drained brown lentils.
- ➢ Simmer for an additional 20-25 minutes, or until the lentils are tender and the stew has thickened slightly.
- ➢ Stir in frozen peas and cook for an additional 2-3 minutes, or until heated through.
- ➢ Season the lentil filling with salt and pepper to taste.

Method (for Mashed Potatoes):
- ➢ While the lentil filling simmers, cook the potatoes in a pot of boiling salted water until tender and easily pierced with a fork.
- ➢ Drain the potatoes and return them to the pot.

Mashing and Seasoning:
- ➢ Using a potato masher, hand mixer, or ricer, mash the potatoes until smooth and creamy.
- ➢ Gradually stir in vegan butter or olive oil and plant-based milk until desired consistency is reached.
- ➢ Season the mashed potatoes with salt and pepper to taste.

Assembling and Baking:
- ➤ Preheat oven to 400°F (200°C).
- ➤ Transfer the lentil filling to a baking dish.
- ➤ Spread the mashed potatoes evenly over the top, creating a smooth and decorative layer.
- ➤ Bake for 20-25 minutes, or until the edges of the mashed potatoes are golden brown and the filling is heated through.

Serving Suggestion:
- ➤ Serve hot with a side of roasted vegetables or a simple green salad.

9. Creamy Vegan Pasta Primavera with Spring Vegetables:

This vibrant pasta dish features fresh spring vegetables tossed in a creamy cashew-based sauce, perfect for a light and flavorful meal.

Ingredients (for Cashew Cream Sauce):
- ➤ 1 cup raw cashews, soaked for at least 2 hours or overnight
- ➤ 1 cup water
- ➤ 1 tablespoon lemon juice
- ➤ 1/4 cup nutritional yeast
- ➤ 1 clove garlic (minced)
- ➤ Salt and pepper to taste

Ingredients (for Pasta Primavera):
- ➤ 12 oz dried pasta (such as penne or farfalle)
- ➤ 1 tablespoon olive oil
- ➤ 1 asparagus bunch (trimmed and chopped)
- ➤ 1 cup sugar snap peas (trimmed and halved)
- ➤ 1 cup cherry tomatoes (halved)

- ➢ 1/2 cup chopped fresh herbs (such as parsley, basil, or mint)
- ➢ Grated vegan parmesan cheese (optional), for garnish

Method (for Cashew Cream Sauce):

- ➢ Drain the soaked cashews and rinse them well.
- ➢ In a blender, combine cashews, water, lemon juice, nutritional yeast, minced garlic, salt, and pepper.
- ➢ Blend until smooth and creamy.
- ➢ You may need to add additional water, a tablespoon at a time, to achieve a desired consistency.

Cooking Pasta and Vegetables:

- ➢ Cook the pasta according to package instructions in a large pot of salted boiling water.
- ➢ While the pasta cooks, heat olive oil in a large skillet over medium heat.
- ➢ Add chopped asparagus and sugar snap peas. Sauté for 5 minutes, or until slightly tender-crisp.
- ➢ Stir in halved cherry tomatoes and cook for an additional minute, or until the tomatoes soften slightly.

Finishing Touches:

- ➢ Drain the cooked pasta and return it to the pot.
- ➢ Add the cashew cream sauce and toss to coat the pasta evenly.
- ➢ Gently fold in the cooked vegetables and chopped fresh herbs.
- ➢ Serve hot with a sprinkle of grated vegan parmesan cheese (optional).

10. Crispy Tofu Tacos with Spicy Mango Salsa (Vegan):

This recipe transforms tofu into a delicious and satisfying taco filling, perfect for a fun and flavorful weeknight meal.

Ingredients (for Spicy Mango Salsa):

- 1 ripe mango (peeled and diced)
- 1/2 red onion (finely chopped)
- 1 jalapeno pepper, seeded and finely chopped (adjust for desired spice level)
- 1/4 cup chopped fresh cilantro
- 1 tablespoon lime juice
- Salt and pepper to taste

Ingredients (for Tofu Tacos):

- 1 block firm tofu (drained and pressed)
- 1/4 cup cornstarch
- 1/4 cup neutral oil (such as canola or vegetable oil)
- 1/2 teaspoon paprika
- 1/4 teaspoon garlic powder
- 1/4 teaspoon onion powder
- Salt and pepper to taste
- Corn tortillas (warmed)
- Vegan sour cream, shredded lettuce, and chopped avocado (optional), for serving

Method (for Spicy Mango Salsa):

- In a medium bowl, combine diced mango, chopped red onion, jalapeno pepper (if using), chopped fresh cilantro, and lime juice.
- Season with salt and pepper to taste.
- Mix well and set aside.

Marinating and Preparing Tofu:

- Cut the drained and pressed tofu into cubes or strips.

> In a shallow dish, toss the tofu cubes with cornstarch to coat evenly.

Cooking the Tofu:
> Heat neutral oil in a large skillet over medium-high heat.
> Add the cornstarch-coated tofu cubes and cook for 5-7 minutes per side, or until golden brown and crispy.
> While the tofu cooks, sprinkle it with paprika, garlic powder, onion powder, salt, and pepper to season.

Assembling the Tacos:
> Warm corn tortillas according to package instructions.
> Fill each tortilla with crispy tofu, spicy mango salsa, vegan sour cream (optional), shredded lettuce, and chopped avocado (optional).

Serving Suggestion:
> Serve immediately and enjoy with your favorite taco toppings!

11. Southwestern Black Bean Burgers with Chipotle Mayo (Vegan):

These hearty and flavorful black bean burgers are perfect for a backyard barbecue or weeknight dinner.

Ingredients (for Black Bean Burgers):
> 1 (15 oz) can black beans, rinsed and drained
> 1 cup cooked brown rice
> 1/2 cup chopped red onion
> 1/4 cup chopped fresh cilantro
> 1 tablespoon olive oil
> 1 tablespoon lime juice
> 1 teaspoon chili powder
> 1/2 teaspoon smoked paprika

- ➢ 1/4 cup breadcrumbs
- ➢ Salt and pepper to taste

Ingredients (for Chipotle Mayo - optional):

- ➢ 1/2 cup vegan mayonnaise
- ➢ 1 chipotle pepper in adobo sauce, chopped (adjust for desired spice level)
- ➢ 1 tablespoon lime juice
- ➢ Salt and pepper to taste

Method (for Black Bean Burgers):

- ➢ In a large bowl, mash together the rinsed and drained black beans with a fork, leaving some texture.
- ➢ Add cooked brown rice, chopped red onion, chopped fresh cilantro, olive oil, lime juice, chili powder, smoked paprika, and breadcrumbs.
- ➢ Season with salt and pepper to taste.
- ➢ Mix well to combine and form into patties.

Cooking the Burgers:

- ➢ Heat a lightly oiled skillet over medium heat.
- ➢ Cook the black bean burgers for 4-5 minutes per side, or until golden brown and heated through.

Chipotle Mayo (Optional):

- ➢ In a small bowl, combine vegan mayonnaise, chopped chipotle pepper in adobo sauce, lime juice, salt, and pepper.
- ➢ Mix well.

Serving Suggestion:

- ➢ Serve the black bean burgers on hamburger buns with your favorite toppings like lettuce, tomato, red onion, avocado, and chipotle mayo (optional).

12. Greek Veggie Moussaka with Lentil "Meat" Sauce (Vegan):

This layered dish features a hearty lentil "meat" sauce, creamy vegan béchamel, and sliced eggplant, creating a flavorful and satisfying Greek-inspired casserole.

Ingredients (for Lentil "Meat" Sauce):

- 2 tablespoons olive oil
- 1 medium onion (chopped)
- 2 cloves garlic (minced)
- 1 carrot, grated
- 1 celery stalk (chopped)
- 1 cup brown lentils (rinsed and drained)
- 4 cups vegetable broth
- 1 (14.5 oz) can diced tomatoes (undrained)
- 1 tablespoon dried oregano
- 1/2 teaspoon ground cumin
- Salt and pepper to taste

Ingredients (for Vegan Béchamel):

- 2 tablespoons vegan butter
- 2 tablespoons all-purpose flour
- 2 cups unsweetened plant-based milk (such as almond milk or soy milk)
- 1/4 cup nutritional yeast
- Salt and pepper to taste

Ingredients (for Assembly):

- 1 large eggplant, thinly sliced
- Olive oil, for brushing
- Vegan grated parmesan cheese (optional), for garnish

Method (for Lentil "Meat" Sauce):

- Heat olive oil in a large pot or Dutch oven over medium heat.
- Add chopped onion, garlic, grated carrot, and chopped celery. Sauté for 5 minutes, or until softened.

- Stir in rinsed and drained brown lentils, vegetable broth, diced tomatoes with their juices, dried oregano, and ground cumin.
- Bring to a boil, then reduce heat and simmer for 30-35 minutes, or until the lentils are tender and the sauce has thickened slightly.
- Season with salt and pepper to taste.

Method (for Vegan Béchamel):

- In a saucepan, melt vegan butter over medium heat.
- Whisk in all-purpose flour and cook for 1 minute, creating a roux.
- Gradually whisk in unsweetened plant-based milk, a little at a time, until a smooth and creamy sauce forms.
- Stir in nutritional yeast, salt, and pepper to season.

Preparing Eggplant:

- Preheat oven to 400°F (200°C).
- Brush eggplant slices with olive oil and arrange them on a baking sheet.
- Bake for 10-15 minutes per side, or until tender and slightly browned.

Assembling and Baking:

- In a baking dish, spread a layer of lentil "meat" sauce.
- Top with a layer of baked eggplant slices.
- Repeat layers, ending with a layer of vegan béchamel sauce.
- Sprinkle with vegan grated parmesan cheese (optional).
- Bake the moussaka for 20-25 minutes, or until heated through and the top is golden brown.

Serving Suggestion:

- Let the moussaka cool slightly before serving.
- Enjoy warm with a side salad or roasted vegetables.

13. **Stuffed Sweet Potato Bowls with Black Beans, Corn, and Avocado Crema (Vegan):**

This colorful and healthy dish features baked sweet potatoes stuffed with a flavorful black bean and corn mixture, topped with a creamy avocado crema.

Ingredients (for Avocado Crema):
- 1 ripe avocado, peeled and pitted
- 1/4 cup chopped fresh cilantro
- 1 tablespoon lime juice
- 1/4 cup water
- Salt and pepper to taste

Ingredients (for Stuffed Sweet Potatoes):
- 2 large sweet potatoes
- 1 tablespoon olive oil
- 1/2 red onion (chopped)
- 1 clove garlic (minced)
- 1 (15 oz) can black beans (rinsed and drained)
- 1 cup frozen corn (thawed)
- 1/2 cup chopped fresh salsa (optional)
- Salt and pepper to taste

Method (for Avocado Crema):
- In a blender or food processor, combine avocado, chopped fresh cilantro, lime juice, and water.
- Blend until smooth and creamy.
- Season with salt and pepper to taste.

Baking Sweet Potatoes:
- Preheat oven to 400°F (200°C).
- Pierce the whole sweet potatoes with a fork a few times.

> ➢ Place them on a baking sheet and bake for 45-60 minutes, or until tender when pierced through with a fork.

Sautéing and Filling:

> ➢ While the sweet potatoes bake, heat olive oil in a large skillet over medium heat.
> ➢ Add chopped red onion and minced garlic.
> ➢ Sauté for 5 minutes, or until softened.
> ➢ Stir in rinsed and drained black beans, thawed corn, and chopped fresh salsa (optional).
> ➢ Season with salt and pepper to taste.
> ➢ Cook for an additional 2-3 minutes, or until heated through.

Assembling and Serving:

> ➢ Once the sweet potatoes are baked, cut them open lengthwise and fluff the flesh slightly with a fork.
> ➢ Fill each sweet potato half with the black bean and corn mixture.
> ➢ Top generously with avocado crema and enjoy!

14. Creamy Vegan Risotto with Butternut Squash and Sage (Vegan):

This comforting risotto features tender arborio rice cooked in a creamy vegan broth with roasted butternut squash and fragrant sage leaves, creating a luxurious and flavorful main course.

Ingredients:

> ➢ 2 tablespoons olive oil
> ➢ 1 medium onion (chopped)
> ➢ 2 cloves garlic (minced)
> ➢ 1 cup arborio rice

- ➢ 4 cups vegetable broth (warmed)
- ➢ 1 cup butternut squash, peeled and diced (roasted or sautéed)
- ➢ 1/2 cup vegan white wine (optional)
- ➢ 1/4 cup chopped fresh sage
- ➢ 1/2 cup grated vegan parmesan cheese (optional)
- ➢ Salt and pepper to taste

Method:

- ➢ Heat olive oil in a large pot or Dutch oven over medium heat.
- ➢ Add chopped onion and minced garlic.
- ➢ Sauté for 5 minutes, or until softened.
- ➢ Stir in the arborio rice and toast for 1 minute, stirring constantly.

Adding Broth and Cooking the Risotto:

- ➢ Add the warmed vegetable broth, one ladleful at a time, allowing the rice to absorb the liquid before adding more.
- ➢ Stir frequently until the rice is creamy and cooked through, about 20-25 minutes.
- ➢ After about 10 minutes of cooking, add the roasted or sautéed butternut squash and vegan white wine (optional).

Finishing Touches:

- ➢ In the last few minutes of cooking, stir in chopped fresh sage and grated vegan parmesan cheese (optional).
- ➢ Season with salt and pepper to taste.

Serving Suggestion:

- ➢ Serve the creamy vegan risotto with butternut squash and sage hot, with additional grated vegan parmesan cheese (optional) for garnish.

15. Thai Coconut Curry Noodle Soup with Vegetables and Tofu (Vegan):

This flavorful and light soup features rice noodles, fresh vegetables, and tofu simmered in a fragrant coconut curry broth, perfect for a comforting and satisfying meal.

Ingredients:
For the Curry Broth:
- 1 tablespoon vegetable oil
- 1 onion, diced
- 2 cloves garlic, minced
- 1 tablespoon Thai red curry paste (adjust for desired spice level)
- 1 teaspoon ground ginger
- 1 (13.5 ounce) can light coconut milk
- 4 cups vegetable broth
- 1 tablespoon soy sauce
- 1 tablespoon brown sugar
- 1 lime, juiced (about 2 tablespoons)
- 1 tablespoon chopped fresh cilantro, plus extra for garnish (optional)

For the Soup:
- 8 ounces block tofu, drained and pressed, cubed
- 1 cup broccoli florets
- 1 red bell pepper (sliced)
- 1 carrot (sliced)
- 8 ounces rice noodles
- Salt and freshly ground black pepper to taste

Preparation:
Prep the Vegetables and Tofu:

> Dice the onion, mince the garlic, slice the red bell pepper and carrot, and break the broccoli florets into bite-sized pieces.
> Drain and press the tofu block, then cut it into cubes.

Methods:

Make the Curry Broth:
> Heat the vegetable oil in a large pot or Dutch oven over medium heat.
> Add the diced onion and cook for 5 minutes, or until softened and translucent.
> Stir in the minced garlic and cook for another minute until fragrant.
> Add the Thai red curry paste and ground ginger, cook for 30 seconds, stirring constantly to release the flavors and toast the spices.
> Pour in the light coconut milk and vegetable broth.
> Stir in the soy sauce, brown sugar, and lime juice.
> Bring to a simmer, then reduce heat to low and simmer for 10 minutes to allow the flavors to meld.

Sauté the Tofu (Optional):
> While the broth simmers, heat a separate pan with a drizzle of oil over medium heat.
> Add the cubed tofu and sauté for 5-7 minutes, or until lightly golden brown on all sides.

Finishing Touches:

Cook the Vegetables:
> Add the broccoli florets, red bell pepper slices, and carrot slices to the simmering broth.
> Cook for 5-7 minutes, or until the vegetables are tender-crisp but still retain a slight bite.

Serving Suggestion:

Cook the Noodles:
> * In a separate pot, cook the rice noodles according to package instructions.
> * Drain and rinse under cold water to stop the cooking process.

Assemble the Soup:
> * Ladle the fragrant coconut curry broth and cooked vegetables into bowls.
> * Add cooked rice noodles and the tofu (if you opted to sauté it).
> * Garnish with a squeeze of lime juice, a sprinkle of freshly ground black pepper, and chopped fresh cilantro (optional).

16. Indian Chickpea Curry with Basmati Rice and Naan (Vegan):

This aromatic curry showcases chickpeas simmered in a rich and flavorful tomato-based sauce with Indian spices, perfect served over basmati rice and fluffy naan bread.

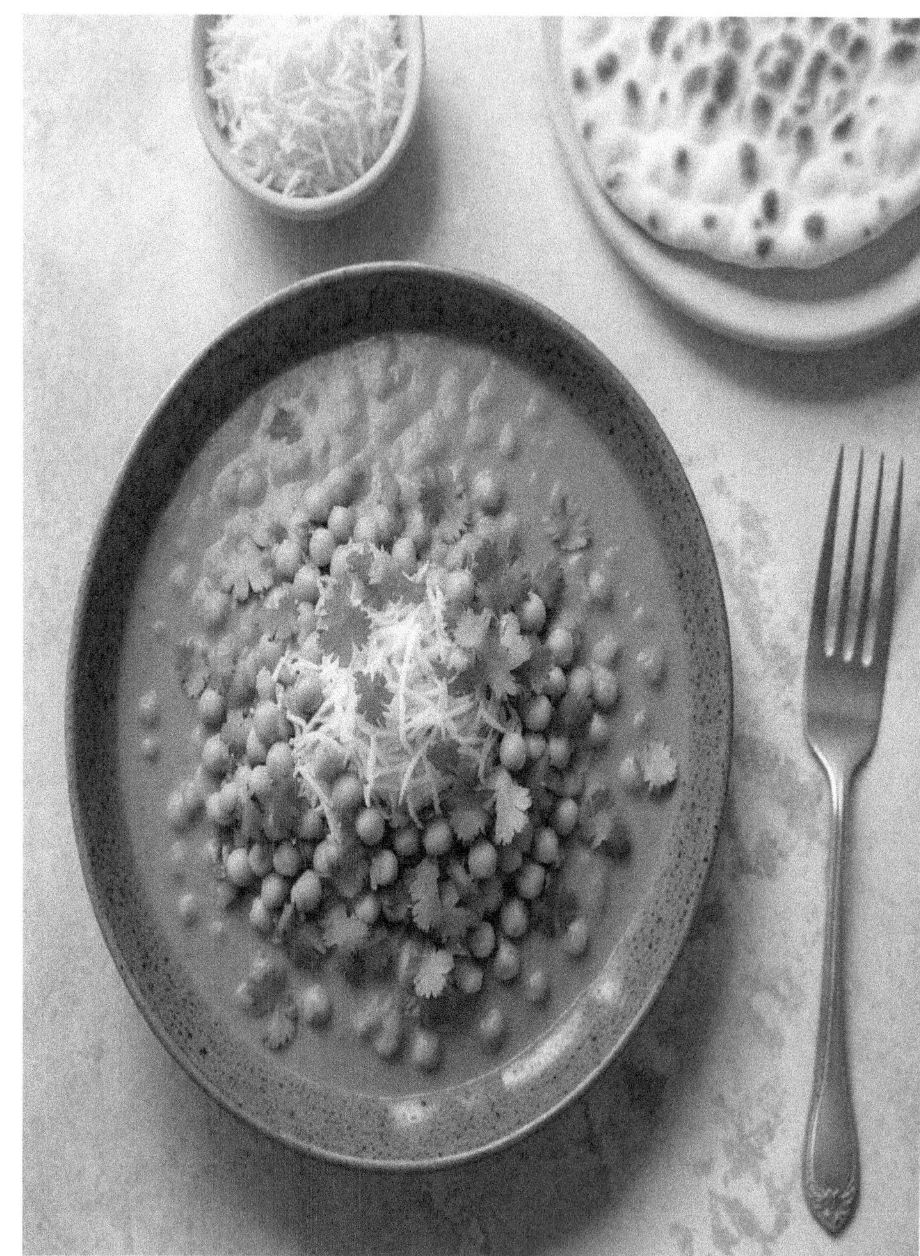

Ingredients:

- ➢ 1 tablespoon vegetable oil
- ➢ 1 medium onion (chopped)
- ➢ 2 cloves garlic (minced)
- ➢ 1 tablespoon grated ginger
- ➢ 1 teaspoon cumin seeds
- ➢ 1/2 teaspoon turmeric powder
- ➢ 1 teaspoon coriander powder
- ➢ 1/2 teaspoon chili powder (adjust for desired spice level)
- ➢ 1 (14.5 oz) can diced tomatoes (undrained)
- ➢ 1 cup vegetable broth
- ➢ 1 (15 oz) can chickpeas (rinsed and drained)
- ➢ 1 cup coconut milk (optional, for a richer flavor)
- ➢ Salt and pepper to taste

Ingredients (for Basmati Rice - optional):

- ➢ 1 cup basmati rice
- ➢ 1 1/2 cups water
- ➢ Salt

Method:

- ➢ Heat vegetable oil in a large pot or Dutch oven over medium heat.
- ➢ Add chopped onion and cook for 5 minutes, or until softened.
- ➢ Stir in minced garlic, grated ginger, cumin seeds, turmeric powder, coriander powder, and chili powder.
- ➢ Cook for an additional minute, allowing the spices to release their aroma.

Adding Liquids and Base:

- ➢ Pour in diced tomatoes with their juices and vegetable broth.

- ➢ Bring to a boil, then reduce heat and simmer for 10 minutes.
- ➢ Stir in rinsed and drained chickpeas and coconut milk (optional).
- ➢ Simmer for an additional 15-20 minutes, or until the chickpeas are tender and the sauce has thickened slightly. Season with salt and pepper to taste.

Cooking Basmati Rice (Optional):
- ➢ In a separate pot, rinse the basmati rice.
- ➢ Combine the rinsed rice with water and a pinch of salt.
- ➢ Bring to a boil, then reduce heat, cover the pot, and simmer for 15-20 minutes, or until the rice is cooked through and fluffy.

Serving Suggestion:
- ➢ Serve the Indian chickpea curry hot over cooked basmati rice (optional) and fluffy naan bread.
- ➢ Garnish with chopped fresh cilantro (optional) for added flavor.

17. Ethiopian Misir Wat (Split Lentil Stew) with Injera (Vegan):

This hearty Ethiopian stew features split lentils simmered in a fragrant berbere spice blend, perfect with injera flatbread for scooping.

Ingredients (for Misir Wat):
- ➢ 2 tablespoons vegetable oil
- ➢ 1 medium onion (chopped)
- ➢ 2 cloves garlic (minced)
- ➢ 1 tablespoon grated ginger
- ➢ 1 tablespoon tomato paste
- ➢ 2 teaspoons berbere spice blend

- ➢ 1 cup red lentils (rinsed and drained)
- ➢ 4 cups vegetable broth
- ➢ Salt and pepper to taste

Ingredients (for Injera - optional):

- ➢ 2 cups teff flour
- ➢ 3/4 cup warm water
- ➢ 1/2 teaspoon sugar
- ➢ Pinch of salt

Method (for Misir Wat):

- ➢ Heat vegetable oil in a large pot or Dutch oven over medium heat.
- ➢ Add chopped onion and cook for 5 minutes, or until softened.
- ➢ Stir in minced garlic, grated ginger, and tomato paste.
- ➢ Cook for an additional minute, allowing the flavors to meld.

Adding Spices and Base:

- ➢ Add berbere spice blend and cook for another minute, until fragrant.
- ➢ Stir in rinsed and drained red lentils, vegetable broth, and salt.
- ➢ Bring to a boil, then reduce heat and simmer for 30-35 minutes, or until the lentils are tender and the stew has thickened slightly.
- ➢ Season with additional salt and pepper to taste.

Injera (Optional):

- ➢ If making injera, combine teff flour, warm water, sugar, and salt in a large bowl.
- ➢ Whisk well until smooth and slightly bubbly.
- ➢ Let the batter rest for at least 2 hours, or preferably overnight, at room temperature.

- ➢ Heat a lightly oiled non-stick skillet or griddle over medium heat.
- ➢ Pour a ladleful of batter onto the skillet and swirl to form a thin crepe-like circle.
- ➢ Cook for 1-2 minutes per side, or until the edges become slightly crisp.
- ➢ Injera should be slightly fermented and have a spongy texture.

Serving Suggestion:
- ➢ Serve the Misir Wat stew spooned onto injera flatbread (if making) or with rice or another grain of your choice.

18. Korean Kimchi Fried Rice with Vegetables and Tofu (Vegan):

This flavorful and quick rice dish features kimchi, vegetables, and pan-fried tofu, creating a satisfying and slightly spicy meal.

Ingredients:
- ➢ 2 tablespoons vegetable oil
- ➢ 1 block firm tofu (drained and cubed)
- ➢ 1/2 cup kimchi (chopped)
- ➢ 1 cup cooked brown rice
- ➢ 1/2 cup mixed vegetables (such as carrots, peas, and corn)
- ➢ 1 tablespoon soy sauce
- ➢ 1 tablespoon rice vinegar
- ➢ 1/2 teaspoon sesame oil
- ➢ Salt and pepper to taste
- ➢ Toasted sesame seeds and chopped scallions, for garnish (optional)

Method:
Heat vegetable oil in a large skillet or wok over medium-high heat. Add the cubed tofu and pan-fry for 5-7 minutes per side, or until

golden brown and crispy. Remove the tofu from the pan and set aside.

Cooking Kimchi and Rice:
- Add the chopped kimchi to the pan and cook for 2-3 minutes, until slightly softened.
- Stir in cooked brown rice and mixed vegetables.
- Pour in soy sauce, rice vinegar, and sesame oil.
- Cook for an additional 3-5 minutes, or until the rice is heated through and the flavors are combined.
- Season with salt and pepper to taste.

Finishing Touches:
- Stir the pan-fried tofu back into the rice mixture.
- Garnish with toasted sesame seeds and chopped scallions (optional) before serving.

19. Moroccan Chickpea Tagine with Sweet Potatoes and Dried Fruits (Vegan):

This aromatic tagine features chickpeas, sweet potatoes, dried fruits, and simmered in a fragrant blend of Moroccan spices, creating a flavorful and satisfying main course.

Ingredients:
- 2 tablespoons olive oil
- 1 medium onion (chopped)
- 2 cloves garlic (minced)
- 1 teaspoon ground ginger
- 1/2 teaspoon turmeric powder
- 1/2 teaspoon cinnamon
- 1/4 teaspoon cumin
- Pinch of saffron threads (optional)
- 1 (14.5 oz) can diced tomatoes, undrained

- ➢ 4 cups vegetable broth
- ➢ 1 cup dried fruits (such as raisins, apricots, and dates)
- ➢ 1 (15 oz) can chickpeas, rinsed and drained
- ➢ 1 large sweet potato, peeled and diced
- ➢ 1/4 cup chopped fresh cilantro
- ➢ Salt and pepper to taste
- ➢ Couscous or crusty bread, for serving (optional)

Method:

- ➢ Heat olive oil in a large pot or Dutch oven over medium heat.
- ➢ Add chopped onion and cook for 5 minutes, or until softened.
- ➢ Stir in minced garlic, ground ginger, turmeric powder, cinnamon, cumin, and saffron threads (if using).
- ➢ Cook for an additional minute, allowing the spices to release their aroma.

Adding Liquids and Base:

- ➢ Pour in diced tomatoes with their juices and vegetable broth.
- ➢ Bring to a boil, then reduce heat and simmer for 10 minutes.
- ➢ Stir in rinsed and drained chickpeas, diced sweet potato, and dried fruits.
- ➢ Simmer for an additional 20-25 minutes, or until the sweet potato is tender and the chickpeas are heated through. Season with salt and pepper to taste.

Finishing Touches:

- ➢ In the last few minutes of cooking, stir in chopped fresh cilantro for added flavor.

Serving Suggestion:

> Serve the Moroccan chickpea tagine with couscous or crusty bread for scooping up the flavorful sauce (optional). Enjoy this warm and comforting dish!

20. Rainbow Veggie Veggie Burgers with Chipotle Mayo (Vegan):

These colorful and flavorful veggie burgers feature a variety of roasted vegetables like grated carrots, beets, and zucchini, creating a healthy and delicious plant-based option.

Ingredients (for Veggie Burgers):
- 1 cup cooked brown rice
- 1/2 cup grated carrots
- 1/2 cup grated beets
- 1/2 cup grated zucchini
- 1/4 cup chopped red onion
- 1/4 cup chopped fresh cilantro
- 1 tablespoon olive oil
- 1 tablespoon lemon juice
- 1/2 teaspoon dried thyme
- 1/4 cup breadcrumbs
- Salt and pepper to taste

Ingredients (for Chipotle Mayo - optional):
- 1/2 cup vegan mayonnaise
- 1 chipotle pepper in adobo sauce, chopped (adjust for desired spice level)
- 1 tablespoon lime juice
- Salt and pepper to taste

Method (for Veggie Burgers):

- ➢ In a large bowl, combine cooked brown rice, grated carrots, beets, and zucchini.
- ➢ Stir in chopped red onion, chopped fresh cilantro, olive oil, lemon juice, dried thyme, and breadcrumbs.
- ➢ Season with salt and pepper to taste.
- ➢ Mix well and form into patties.

Cooking the Burgers:
- ➢ Heat a lightly oiled skillet over medium heat.
- ➢ Cook the veggie burgers for 5-7 minutes per side, or until golden brown and heated through.

Chipotle Mayo (Optional):
- ➢ In a small bowl, combine vegan mayonnaise, chopped chipotle pepper in adobo sauce, lime juice, salt, and pepper.
- ➢ Mix well.

Serving Suggestion:
- ➢ Serve the rainbow veggie burgers on hamburger buns with your favorite toppings like lettuce, tomato, red onion, avocado, and chipotle mayo (optional).

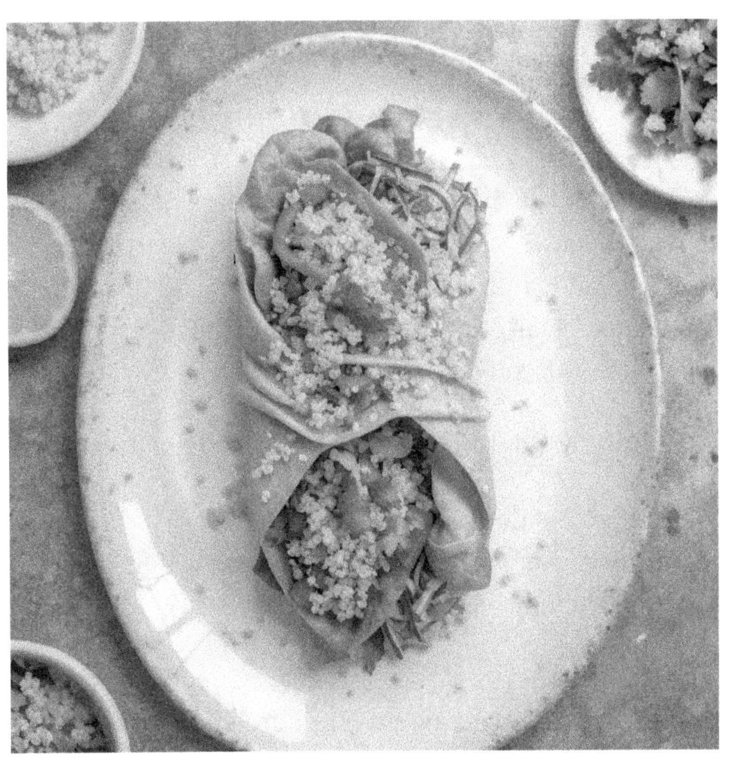

Chapter Four
Vibrant Sides & Salads

Salads and side dishes are often relegated to afterthoughts, but they have the power to transform a simple meal into a symphony of flavors and textures. This chapter dives into a world of vibrant and delicious plant-based options, ensuring every plate is not just complete, but truly exciting.

1. Rainbow Roasted Vegetables with Balsamic Glaze:

This classic side dish takes center stage with a stunning array of colorful vegetables, caramelized to perfection and drizzled with a sweet and tangy balsamic glaze.

Ingredients:
- 1 head broccoli (cut into florets)
- 1 red bell pepper (sliced)
- 1 yellow bell pepper (sliced)
- 1 red onion, cut into wedges
- 1 zucchini (sliced)
- 1 tablespoon olive oil
- Salt and pepper to taste

For the Balsamic Glaze:
- 1/2 cup balsamic vinegar
- 1 tablespoon brown sugar
- 1 teaspoon cornstarch (optional, for a thicker glaze)

Method:
- Preheat oven to 400°F (200°C).
- Line a baking sheet with parchment paper.

- ➢ In a large bowl, toss the broccoli florets, sliced bell peppers, red onion wedges, and zucchini slices with olive oil, salt, and pepper.
- ➢ Ensure everything is evenly coated.
- ➢ Spread the vegetables on the prepared baking sheet in a single layer.
- ➢ Roast for 20-25 minutes, or until the vegetables are tender-crisp and slightly browned at the edges.

Making the Balsamic Glaze (Optional):
- ➢ While the vegetables roast, in a small saucepan, combine balsamic vinegar and brown sugar.
- ➢ Heat over medium heat, stirring occasionally, until the mixture thickens and becomes syrupy. This takes about 5-7 minutes.
- ➢ If you prefer a thicker glaze, whisk a teaspoon of cornstarch with a tablespoon of water to create a slurry.
- ➢ Stir the slurry into the simmering balsamic mixture and cook for an additional minute, or until the glaze thickens to your desired consistency.

Serving Suggestion:
- ➢ Once the vegetables are roasted, arrange them on a serving platter.
- ➢ Drizzle with the balsamic glaze (optional) and enjoy!

2. Creamy Vegan Tzatziki with Fresh Herbs:

This cool and refreshing dip is the perfect accompaniment to crudités, pita bread, or even dolloped on top of roasted vegetables or falafel.

Ingredients:
- 1 cup unsweetened plain plant-based yogurt (such as soy yogurt or coconut yogurt)
- 1 medium cucumber (grated)
- 1 tablespoon chopped fresh dill
- 1 tablespoon chopped fresh mint
- 1 tablespoon lemon juice
- 1 clove garlic (minced)
- Salt and pepper to taste

Method:
- In a medium bowl, whisk together unsweetened plant-based yogurt, grated cucumber, chopped fresh dill, chopped fresh mint, lemon juice, minced garlic, salt, and pepper.
- Cover the bowl and refrigerate for at least 30 minutes to allow the flavors to meld. The tzatziki will thicken slightly as it chills.

Serving Suggestion:

Serve the creamy vegan tzatziki with fresh herbs alongside crudités like carrot sticks, celery sticks, cucumber slices, or pita bread for dipping. It's also delicious drizzled over falafel or roasted vegetables.

3. Quinoa Salad with Roasted Butternut Squash and Cranberries:

This protein-packed salad features fluffy quinoa tossed with roasted butternut squash, tart cranberries, and a light and flavorful vinaigrette.

Ingredients:
- 1 cup quinoa, rinsed
- 1 ½ cups vegetable broth
- 1 medium butternut squash, peeled and diced

- ➢ 1 tablespoon olive oil
- ➢ 1/2 cup dried cranberries
- ➢ 1/4 cup chopped fresh parsley
- ➢ Salt and pepper to taste

For the Vinaigrette:

- ➢ 2 tablespoons olive oil
- ➢ 1 tablespoon apple cider vinegar
- ➢ 1 tablespoon lemon juice
- ➢ 1 teaspoon Dijon mustard
- ➢ Salt and pepper to taste

Method (for Cooking Quinoa):

- ➢ In a saucepan, combine rinsed quinoa with vegetable broth.
- ➢ Bring to a boil, then reduce heat, cover, and simmer for 15-20 minutes, or until the quinoa is cooked through and fluffy.
- ➢ Remove from heat and let fluff with a fork for 5 minutes.

Roasting Butternut Squash:

- ➢ Preheat oven to 400°F (200°C).
- ➢ Toss the diced butternut squash with olive oil and season with salt and pepper.
- ➢ Spread the diced squash on a baking sheet in a single layer and roast for 20-25 minutes, or until tender and slightly browned at the edges.

Assembling the Salad:

- ➢ In a large bowl, combine the cooked quinoa, roasted butternut squash, dried cranberries, and chopped fresh parsley.

Making the Vinaigrette:

- ➢ In a small bowl, whisk together olive oil, apple cider vinegar, lemon juice, Dijon mustard, salt, and pepper.

Finishing Touches:

- ➢ Pour the vinaigrette over the salad ingredients and toss to coat everything evenly.
- ➢ Season with additional salt and pepper to taste (optional).

Serving Suggestion:

- ➢ Serve the quinoa salad with roasted butternut squash and cranberries at room temperature or chilled. It's a perfect accompaniment to grilled tofu, tempeh, or lentil burgers.

4. Massaged Kale Salad with Lemon Tahini Dressing:

This vibrant salad features massaged kale leaves for a tender texture, tossed with a bright and tangy lemon tahini dressing.

Ingredients:

- ➢ 1 bunch kale, ribs removed and leaves roughly chopped
- ➢ 1/2 cup cherry tomatoes, halved
- ➢ 1/4 cup crumbled vegan feta cheese (optional)
- ➢ 1/4 cup chopped walnuts or pecans

For the Lemon Tahini Dressing:

- ➢ 2 tablespoons tahini
- ➢ 2 tablespoons olive oil
- ➢ 1 tablespoon lemon juice
- ➢ 1 tablespoon water
- ➢ 1 clove garlic (minced)
- ➢ 1/2 teaspoon dried dill
- ➢ Salt and pepper to taste

Method (for Massaging Kale):

- ➢ In a large bowl, place the chopped kale leaves.
- ➢ Drizzle with a tablespoon of olive oil and sprinkle with a pinch of salt.

- ➢ Using your hands, massage the kale leaves for several minutes until they become wilted and tender.
- ➢ This process helps break down the tough fibers in kale, making it more palatable.

Assembling the Salad:

- ➢ Once the kale is massaged, add the halved cherry tomatoes, crumbled vegan feta cheese (optional), and chopped walnuts or pecans to the bowl.

Making the Lemon Tahini Dressing:

- ➢ In a small bowl, whisk together tahini, olive oil, lemon juice, water, minced garlic, dried dill, salt, and pepper.

Finishing Touches:

- ➢ Pour the lemon tahini dressing over the salad ingredients and toss to coat everything evenly.
- ➢ Season with additional salt and pepper to taste (optional).

Serving Suggestion:

- ➢ Serve the massaged kale salad with lemon tahini dressing immediately. It's a light and refreshing side dish or a healthy lunch option.

5. Asian-Inspired Slaw with Peanut Dressing:

This colorful slaw features shredded vegetables like cabbage, carrots, and bell peppers, tossed in a flavorful peanut dressing with a hint of sweetness and spice.

Ingredients:

- ➢ 3 cups shredded green cabbage
- ➢ 1 cup shredded carrots
- ➢ 1/2 cup chopped red bell pepper
- ➢ 1/4 cup chopped green onions

For the Peanut Dressing:

- 1/4 cup peanut butter (creamy or chunky)
- 2 tablespoons soy sauce (low-sodium preferred)
- 1 tablespoon rice vinegar
- 1 tablespoon honey or maple syrup
- 1 tablespoon sriracha (adjust for desired spice level)
- 1 tablespoon lime juice
- 1 clove garlic, minced
- 1/4 cup water

Method (for Shredding Vegetables):

- Using a mandoline slicer or a sharp knife, shred the green cabbage, carrots, and red bell pepper.
- Thinly slice the green onions.

Making the Peanut Dressing:

- In a small bowl, whisk together peanut butter, soy sauce, rice vinegar, honey or maple syrup, sriracha, lime juice, minced garlic, and water.
- The dressing should be creamy yet pourable. You may need to add additional water, a tablespoon at a time, to achieve the desired consistency.

Assembling the Salad:

- In a large bowl, combine the shredded cabbage, carrots, red bell pepper, and chopped green onions.

Adding the Dressing:

- Pour the peanut dressing over the salad ingredients and toss to coat everything evenly.
- Season with additional salt and pepper to taste (optional).

Serving Suggestion:

- Serve the Asian-inspired slaw with peanut dressing chilled or at room temperature. It's a perfect accompaniment to grilled tofu, tempeh, or Asian-inspired noodle dishes.

6. Roasted Brussels Sprouts with Balsamic Glaze and Pecans:

Brussels sprouts get a delicious makeover with this recipe. Roasting caramelizes the natural sweetness of the sprouts, while the balsamic glaze adds a touch of tang. Toasted pecans provide a delightful crunch.

Ingredients:
- 1 pound Brussels sprouts, trimmed and halved
- 1 tablespoon olive oil
- Salt and pepper to taste
- 1/4 cup chopped pecans

For the Balsamic Glaze (see recipe in Rainbow Roasted Vegetables - Chapter 4, recipe 1):

Follow the recipe for balsamic glaze mentioned in Chapter 4, recipe 1 (Rainbow Roasted Vegetables). You can adjust the amount of balsamic vinegar and brown sugar depending on your desired glaze quantity.

Method (for Roasting Brussels Sprouts):
- Preheat oven to 400°F (200°C).
- Line a baking sheet with parchment paper.
- In a large bowl, toss the halved Brussels sprouts with olive oil, salt, and pepper.
- Ensure everything is evenly coated.
- Spread the Brussels sprouts on the prepared baking sheet in a single layer.
- Roast for 20-25 minutes, or until the Brussels sprouts are tender-crisp and slightly browned at the edges.

Toasting Pecans:
- While the Brussels sprouts roast, heat a small skillet over medium heat.

- ➢ Add the chopped pecans and toast for a few minutes, stirring occasionally, until fragrant and lightly golden brown.
- ➢ Watch closely to prevent burning.

Assembling the Dish:
- ➢ Once the Brussels sprouts are roasted, remove them from the oven and transfer them to a serving dish.
- ➢ Drizzle the balsamic glaze over the roasted Brussels sprouts (use the amount you prefer).
- ➢ Sprinkle the toasted pecans on top for added texture and flavor.

Serving Suggestion:
- ➢ Serve the roasted Brussels sprouts with balsamic glaze and pecans warm. This flavorful side dish complements roasted chicken, tempeh, or lentil loaf.

7. Creamy Vegan Mac and Cheese with Hidden Vegetables:

This dish is a crowd-pleaser! A creamy cashew-based sauce coats elbow macaroni, while hidden pureed vegetables like cauliflower or butternut squash add a sneaky dose of nutrients.

Ingredients:
- ➢ 1 cup raw cashews, soaked in hot water for at least 1 hour
- ➢ 1 cup unsweetened plant-based milk (such as almond milk or cashew milk)
- ➢ 1 tablespoon nutritional yeast
- ➢ 1 tablespoon lemon juice
- ➢ 1 tablespoon olive oil
- ➢ 1 clove garlic (minced)
- ➢ 1 cup cooked and chopped cauliflower florets (or butternut squash)

- ➢ 10 oz elbow macaroni (or other preferred pasta shape)
- ➢ 1/2 cup vegan cheddar cheese shreds (optional)
- ➢ Salt and pepper to taste

Method (for Cashew Sauce):

- ➢ Drain the soaked cashews and rinse briefly with fresh water
- ➢ Add the cashews, unsweetened plant-based milk, nutritional yeast, lemon juice, olive oil, minced garlic, and salt to a blender.
- ➢ Blend until smooth and creamy.
- ➢ You may need to add additional water, a tablespoon at a time, to achieve a pourable consistency.

Cooking Vegetables (for hidden veggies):

- ➢ While the cashews soak, steam or boil the cauliflower florets (or butternut squash) until tender.
- ➢ Once cooked, puree the vegetables in a blender or food processor until smooth.

Cooking Pasta:

- ➢ Cook the elbow macaroni according to package instructions in a large pot of boiling water.
- ➢ Drain and set aside.

Assembling the Mac and Cheese:

- ➢ In a large pot or saucepan, combine the creamy cashew sauce and pureed vegetables (cauliflower or butternut squash).
- ➢ Heat over medium heat, stirring occasionally, until warmed through. Season with additional salt and pepper to taste.
- ➢ Add the cooked and drained elbow macaroni to the sauce and toss to coat everything evenly.
- ➢ If using, sprinkle the vegan cheddar cheese shreds on top of the mac and cheese (optional).

Baking (optional):

- ➢ Preheat oven to broil.
- ➢ For a cheesy topping, transfer the mac and cheese to a baking dish and broil for a few minutes, or until the top is slightly golden brown.
- ➢ Watch closely to prevent burning.

Serving Suggestion:
- ➢ Serve the creamy vegan mac and cheese with hidden vegetables warm. It's a comforting and satisfying side dish or a delicious main course on its own.

8. Spicy Edamame with Garlic and Chili Flakes:

This protein-packed snack or side dish is quick and easy to prepare. Edamame pods are tossed with olive oil, garlic, and chili flakes for a satisfying and flavorful treat.

Ingredients:
- ➢ 1 package frozen edamame (shelled or in pods)
- ➢ 1 tablespoon olive oil
- ➢ 2 cloves garlic (minced)
- ➢ 1/2 teaspoon chili flakes (adjust for desired spice level)
- ➢ Salt and pepper to taste

Method:
- ➢ Cook the edamame according to package instructions.
- ➢ If using frozen edamame in pods, blanch them in boiling water for 3-5 minutes, or until tender-crisp.
- ➢ Drain and remove the edamame from the pods (optional).

Sautéing Garlic and Chili Flakes:
- ➢ While the edamame cooks, heat olive oil in a large skillet or pan over medium heat.

- Add the minced garlic and cook for 30 seconds, or until fragrant.
- Be careful not to burn the garlic.

Adding Edamame and Seasonings:

- Add the cooked edamame (shelled or in pods) to the pan with the garlic.
- Toss to coat the edamame with the olive oil and garlic.
- Sprinkle the chili flakes over the edamame and toss again.
- Adjust the amount of chili flakes depending on your desired spice level.

Finishing Touches:

- Season with salt and pepper to taste.
- Cook for an additional minute or two, stirring occasionally, to allow the flavors to meld.

Serving Suggestion:

- Serve the spicy edamame with garlic and chili flakes warm or at room temperature. It's a perfect appetizer, snack, or addition to a lunchbox.

9. Rainbow Veggie Skewers with Chimichurri Sauce:

These colorful veggie skewers are perfect for grilling or pan-frying. Bell peppers, zucchini, onions, and cherry tomatoes are threaded onto skewers and cooked until tender-crisp. A vibrant chimichurri sauce adds a burst of freshness.

Ingredients:

- 1 red bell pepper, cut into squares
- 1 yellow bell pepper, cut into squares
- 1 zucchini, cut into thick slices
- 1 red onion, cut into wedges
- 1 pint cherry tomatoes

> Wooden skewers (soaked in water for at least 30 minutes to prevent burning)

For the Chimichurri Sauce:
> 1 cup fresh parsley leaves, chopped
> 1/4 cup fresh cilantro leaves, chopped
> 2 cloves garlic, minced
> 1/4 cup olive oil
> 2 tablespoons red wine vinegar
> 1/2 teaspoon dried oregano
> Salt and pepper to taste

Method (for Assembling Skewers):
> Thread the bell pepper squares, zucchini slices, red onion wedges, and cherry tomatoes onto the soaked wooden skewers, alternating colors for visual appeal.
> Ensure the vegetables are not overcrowded on the skewers.

Cooking the Skewers:
> You can grill the skewers on a preheated outdoor grill or pan-fry them in a large skillet with a drizzle of olive oil over medium heat.
> Cook the skewers for 5-7 minutes per side, or until the vegetables are tender-crisp and slightly charred.

Making the Chimichurri Sauce:
> In a food processor or blender, combine chopped fresh parsley, chopped fresh cilantro, minced garlic, olive oil, red wine vinegar, dried oregano, salt, and pepper.
> Pulse until a chunky sauce forms.
> You can adjust the consistency by adding more olive oil if desired.

Serving Suggestion:

> Serve the rainbow veggie skewers warm with a generous drizzle of chimichurri sauce on the side. This dish is a light and flavorful side dish or a vegetarian main course.

10. Marinated Artichoke Hearts with Herbs and Lemon:

Marinated artichoke hearts are a delightful appetizer or side dish. This recipe features artichoke hearts marinated in a flavorful blend of olive oil, lemon juice, herbs, and garlic, resulting in a tangy and delicious accompaniment for any meal.

Ingredients:
- 1 jar marinated artichoke hearts (drained)
- 1/4 cup olive oil
- 2 tablespoons lemon juice
- 1 tablespoon chopped fresh parsley
- 1 tablespoon chopped fresh thyme
- 1 clove garlic, minced
- Salt and pepper to taste

Method:
- In a bowl, combine olive oil, lemon juice, chopped fresh parsley, chopped fresh thyme, minced garlic, salt, and pepper.
- Whisk the ingredients together to create a marinade.

Marinating the Artichoke Hearts:
- Add the drained artichoke hearts to the marinade mixture.
- Toss to coat the artichoke hearts evenly.
- Cover the bowl and refrigerate for at least 30 minutes, or up to overnight, to allow the flavors to develop.

Serving Suggestion:
- Serve the marinated artichoke hearts chilled or at room temperature.

- They can be enjoyed on their own as an appetizer, or spooned over a bed of greens for a light and flavorful salad.
- You can also use marinated artichoke hearts to add a tangy twist to pizzas, pastas, or grain bowls.

11. Moroccan Carrot Salad with Cherries and Almonds:

This refreshing salad features julienned carrots tossed with a fragrant Moroccan-inspired dressing, studded with sweet cherries and crunchy almonds.

Ingredients:
- 3 cups carrots, julienned
- 1/2 cup dried cherries
- 1/4 cup sliced almonds
- Fresh cilantro, for garnish (optional)

For the Moroccan Dressing:
- 2 tablespoons olive oil
- 1 tablespoon lemon juice
- 1 tablespoon orange juice
- 1 teaspoon ground cumin
- 1/2 teaspoon ground coriander
- Pinch of cinnamon
- Salt and pepper to taste

Method (for Dressing):
- In a small bowl, whisk together olive oil, lemon juice, orange juice, ground cumin, ground coriander, cinnamon, salt, and pepper.

Assembling the Salad:
- In a large bowl, combine the julienned carrots, dried cherries, and sliced almonds.
- Pour the Moroccan dressing over the salad ingredients and toss to coat everything evenly.

Serving Suggestion:

- Serve the Moroccan carrot salad with cherries and almonds chilled or at room temperature. Garnish with fresh cilantro (optional) for a pop of color and additional flavor.

12. Edamame and Corn Succotash with Herbs:

This vibrant side dish combines fresh or frozen edamame, sweet corn kernels, and chopped herbs for a simple yet flavorful accompaniment.

Ingredients:

- 1 cup shelled edamame (fresh or frozen)
- 1 cup fresh corn kernels (or frozen corn)
- 1/4 cup chopped fresh parsley
- 1 tablespoon olive oil
- Salt and pepper to taste

Method (for Cooking Edamame):

- If using fresh edamame, blanch them in boiling water for 3-5 minutes, or until tender-crisp.
- Drain and remove the edamame from the pods (optional).
- Frozen edamame can be cooked according to package instructions.

Cooking Corn:

- If using fresh corn, blanch the corn kernels in boiling water for 2-3 minutes, or until tender.
- Drain and set aside. Frozen corn can be cooked according to package instructions.

Combining Ingredients:

- In a large bowl, combine cooked edamame, corn kernels, and chopped fresh parsley.
- Drizzle with olive oil and season with salt and pepper to taste.
- Toss to coat everything evenly.

Serving Suggestion:

> ➤ Serve the edamame and corn succotash with herbs warm or at room temperature. It's a perfect accompaniment to grilled tofu, tempeh, or lentil burgers.

13. Roasted Sweet Potato Salad with Black Beans and Avocado:

Roasted sweet potatoes add a touch of sweetness to this hearty salad, balanced by black beans and creamy avocado.

Ingredients:
> ➤ 1 medium sweet potato (peeled and diced)
> ➤ 1 tablespoon olive oil
> ➤ 1/2 teaspoon ground cumin
> ➤ 1/4 teaspoon chili powder (optional)
> ➤ Salt and pepper to taste
> ➤ 1 (15 oz) can black beans (rinsed and drained)
> ➤ 1 ripe avocado (diced)
> ➤ 1/4 cup chopped fresh cilantro
> ➤ Lime wedges, for serving

Method (for Roasting Sweet Potato):
> ➤ Preheat oven to 400°F (200°C).
> ➤ Line a baking sheet with parchment paper.
> ➤ In a large bowl, toss the diced sweet potato with olive oil, ground cumin, chili powder (optional), salt, and pepper.
> ➤ Ensure everything is evenly coated.
> ➤ Spread the sweet potato on the prepared baking sheet in a single layer.
> ➤ Roast for 20-25 minutes, or until the sweet potato is tender and slightly browned at the edges.

Assembling the Salad:
> ➤ Once roasted, let the sweet potato cool slightly.
> ➤ In a large bowl, combine the roasted sweet potato, rinsed and drained black beans, diced avocado, and chopped fresh cilantro.

Serving Suggestion:
> - Serve the roasted sweet potato salad with black beans and avocado at room temperature.
> - Squeeze fresh lime wedges over the salad for an added touch of acidity before serving.

14. Spicy Thai Mango Salad with Peanuts:

This vibrant salad features julienned green mangoes tossed in a spicy Thai dressing with crunchy peanuts and fresh herbs.

Ingredients:
> - 1 unripe green mango (julienned)
> - 1/2 cup chopped red onion
> - 1/4 cup chopped fresh cilantro
> - 1/4 cup chopped fresh mint
> - 2 tablespoons roasted peanuts (chopped)

For the Spicy Thai Dressing:
> - 2 tablespoons lime juice
> - 1 tablespoon fish sauce (vegetarian option: substitute with soy sauce)
> - 1 tablespoon brown sugar
> - 1 tablespoon vegetable oil
> - 1 clove garlic (minced)
> - 1/2 teaspoon red chili flakes (adjust for desired spice level)

Method (for Dressing):
> - In a small bowl, whisk together lime juice, fish sauce (or soy sauce), brown sugar, vegetable oil, minced garlic, and red chili flakes.

Assembling the Salad:
> - In a large bowl, combine the julienned green mango, chopped red onion, chopped fresh cilantro, and chopped fresh mint.
> - Pour the spicy Thai dressing over the salad ingredients and toss to coat everything evenly.

Finishing Touches:
> ➢ Sprinkle the chopped roasted peanuts on top of the salad just before serving.

Serving Suggestion:
> ➢ Serve the spicy Thai mango salad with peanuts chilled or at room temperature. It's a refreshing and flavorful side dish or a light lunch option.

15. Grilled Halloumi with Watermelon and Mint Salad:

Salty grilled halloumi cheese pairs perfectly with sweet and juicy watermelon chunks in this refreshing summer salad.

Ingredients:
> ➢ 1/2 block halloumi cheese, sliced into 1/2-inch thick slices
> ➢ 1 tablespoon olive oil
> ➢ 3 cups cubed seedless watermelon
> ➢ 1/4 cup fresh mint leaves, chopped
> ➢ Salt and pepper to taste

Method (for Grilling Halloumi):
> ➢ Heat a grill pan or skillet over medium heat.
> ➢ Brush the halloumi slices with olive oil.
> ➢ Grill the halloumi for 2-3 minutes per side, or until golden brown and slightly softened.

Assembling the Salad:
> ➢ In a large bowl, combine the cubed watermelon and chopped fresh mint leaves.

Serving Suggestion:
> ➢ Arrange the grilled halloumi slices on top of the watermelon salad.
> ➢ Season with salt and pepper to taste (optional).
> ➢ Serve immediately while the halloumi is still warm.

16. Creamy Coconut Curry Lentil Salad:

This protein-packed salad features cooked lentils tossed in a flavorful coconut curry sauce, perfect for a satisfying and healthy side dish.

Ingredients:
- 1 cup brown lentils, rinsed and cooked
- 1 (13.5 oz) can coconut milk
- 1 tablespoon curry powder
- 1 tablespoon yellow curry paste (optional, for more intense flavor)
- 1 tablespoon soy sauce
- 1 tablespoon lime juice
- 1/2 cup chopped red bell pepper
- 1/4 cup chopped green onion
- Cilantro leaves, for garnish (optional)

Method (for Cooking Lentils):
- In a pot, rinse the brown lentils. Cover them with water and bring to a boil. Reduce heat and simmer for 20-25 minutes, or until lentils are tender but still hold their shape.
- Drain and set aside.

Making the Coconut Curry Sauce:
- In a saucepan, whisk together coconut milk, curry powder, yellow curry paste (optional), soy sauce, and lime juice.
- Heat over medium heat until simmering.

Assembling the Salad:
- In a large bowl, combine the cooked lentils, chopped red bell pepper, and chopped green onion.
- Pour the warm coconut curry sauce over the salad ingredients and toss to coat everything evenly.

Serving Suggestion:

- ➢ Serve the creamy coconut curry lentil salad warm or at room temperature.
- ➢ Garnish with fresh cilantro leaves (optional) for an extra pop of color and flavor.

17. Quinoa Tabbouleh with Fresh Herbs and Lemon:

This vibrant salad takes a twist on the classic tabbouleh recipe, featuring quinoa instead of bulgur wheat and a refreshing lemon dressing.

Ingredients:
- ➢ 1 cup quinoa, rinsed
- ➢ 2 cups boiling water
- ➢ 1 cup chopped cucumber
- ➢ 1 cup chopped cherry tomatoes
- ➢ 1/2 cup chopped fresh parsley
- ➢ 1/4 cup chopped fresh mint
- ➢ 2 tablespoons olive oil
- ➢ 1 tablespoon lemon juice
- ➢ Salt and pepper to taste

Method (for Cooking Quinoa):
- ➢ In a saucepan, combine rinsed quinoa and boiling water.
- ➢ Bring to a boil, then reduce heat, cover, and simmer for 15-20 minutes, or until the quinoa is cooked through and fluffy.
- ➢ Fluff the quinoa with a fork and set aside to cool slightly.

Assembling the Salad:
- ➢ In a large bowl, combine the cooked quinoa, chopped cucumber, chopped cherry tomatoes, chopped fresh parsley, and chopped fresh mint.

Making the Lemon Dressing:
- ➢ In a small bowl, whisk together olive oil, lemon juice, salt, and pepper.

Finishing Touches:

- ➢ Pour the lemon dressing over the salad ingredients and toss to coat everything evenly.
- ➢ Season with additional salt and pepper to taste (optional).

Serving Suggestion:
- ➢ Serve the quinoa tabbouleh with fresh herbs and lemon chilled or at room temperature. It's a light and refreshing side dish or a perfect lunch option.

18. Roasted Butternut Squash with Sage and Maple Glaze:

This recipe offers a delicious twist on roasted vegetables. Butternut squash cubes are tossed with sage leaves and roasted until tender, then glazed with a sweet and savory maple glaze.

Ingredients:
- ➢ 1 medium butternut squash, peeled and cubed
- ➢ 1 tablespoon olive oil
- ➢ 1/2 teaspoon dried sage
- ➢ Salt and pepper to taste

For the Maple Glaze:
- ➢ 1/4 cup pure maple syrup
- ➢ 1 tablespoon balsamic vinegar
- ➢ 1 teaspoon Dijon mustard

Method (for Roasting Butternut Squash):
- ➢ Preheat oven to 400°F (200°C).
- ➢ Line a baking sheet with parchment paper.
- ➢ In a large bowl, toss the cubed butternut squash with olive oil, dried sage, salt, and pepper.
- ➢ Ensure everything is evenly coated.
- ➢ Spread the butternut squash on the prepared baking sheet in a single layer.

➤ Roast for 20-25 minutes, or until the squash is tender and slightly browned at the edges.

Making the Maple Glaze:
➤ In a small saucepan, whisk together pure maple syrup, balsamic vinegar, and Dijon mustard.
➤ Heat over medium heat until the glaze thickens slightly, stirring occasionally.

Finishing Touches:
➤ Once the butternut squash is roasted, remove it from the oven and drizzle with the prepared maple glaze.
➤ Toss to coat the squash cubes evenly.
➤ Broil the glazed butternut squash for an additional 1-2 minutes, or until the glaze becomes slightly caramelized. Watch closely to prevent burning.

Serving Suggestion:
➤ Serve the roasted butternut squash with sage and maple glaze warm.
➤ It's a flavorful and comforting side dish that complements roasted tempeh, lentils, or quinoa.

19. Rainbow Power Slaw with Tahini Dressing:

This colorful slaw features shredded cabbage, carrots, and other colorful vegetables tossed in a creamy tahini dressing.

Ingredients:
➤ 3 cups shredded green cabbage
➤ 1 cup shredded carrots
➤ 1/2 cup chopped red bell pepper
➤ 1/4 cup chopped green onion
➤ 1/4 cup chopped fresh cilantro
➤ Additional vegetables for extra color (optional): shredded broccoli slaw, chopped jicama, or thinly sliced radishes

For the Tahini Dressing:

- ➤ 1/3 cup tahini
- ➤ 2 tablespoons lemon juice
- ➤ 2 tablespoons water
- ➤ 1 tablespoon olive oil
- ➤ 1 clove garlic (minced)
- ➤ 1/2 teaspoon ground cumin
- ➤ Salt and pepper to taste

Method (for Dressing):

- ➤ In a blender or food processor, combine tahini, lemon juice, water, olive oil, minced garlic, ground cumin, salt, and pepper. Blend until smooth and creamy. You may need to add additional water, a tablespoon at a time, to achieve a desired pouring consistency.

Assembling the Salad:

- ➤ In a large bowl, combine the shredded green cabbage, shredded carrots, chopped red bell pepper, chopped green onion, chopped fresh cilantro, and any additional chopped vegetables you'd like to include (broccoli slaw, jicama, or radishes).

Serving Suggestion:

- ➤ Pour the creamy tahini dressing over the salad ingredients and toss to coat everything evenly.
- ➤ Serve the rainbow power slaw with tahini dressing chilled or at room temperature. It's a refreshing and flavorful side dish or a light lunch option.

20. Asian Noodle Salad with Peanut Sauce:

This flavorful salad features rice noodles, fresh vegetables, and a tangy peanut sauce, perfect for a satisfying and light meal.

Ingredients:

- ➤ 8 oz rice noodles (such as thin rice vermicelli)
- ➤ 2 cups shredded vegetables (such as carrots, cucumbers, and red bell pepper)

> 1/2 cup chopped fresh cilantro
> Peanuts, chopped, for garnish (optional)

For the Peanut Sauce:

> 1/3 cup peanut butter (creamy or chunky)
> 2 tablespoons soy sauce (low-sodium preferred)
> 1 tablespoon rice vinegar
> 1 tablespoon honey or maple syrup
> 1 tablespoon sriracha (adjust for desired spice level)
> 1 tablespoon lime juice
> 1 clove garlic (minced)
> 1/4 cup water

Method (for Cooking Rice Noodles):

> Cook the rice noodles according to package instructions. Drain and rinse under cold water to stop the cooking process.

Making the Peanut Sauce:

> In a small bowl, whisk together peanut butter, soy sauce, rice vinegar, honey or maple syrup, sriracha, lime juice, minced garlic, and water. The sauce should be creamy yet pourable. You may need to adjust the consistency by adding more water or peanut butter.

Assembling the Salad:

> In a large bowl, combine the cooked and rinsed rice noodles, shredded vegetables, and chopped fresh cilantro.

Finishing Touches:

> Pour the peanut sauce over the salad ingredients and toss to coat everything evenly. Garnish with chopped peanuts (optional) before serving.

Serving Suggestion:

> Serve the Asian noodle salad with peanut sauce chilled or at room temperature. It's a refreshing and flavorful salad, perfect for a light lunch or a side dish.

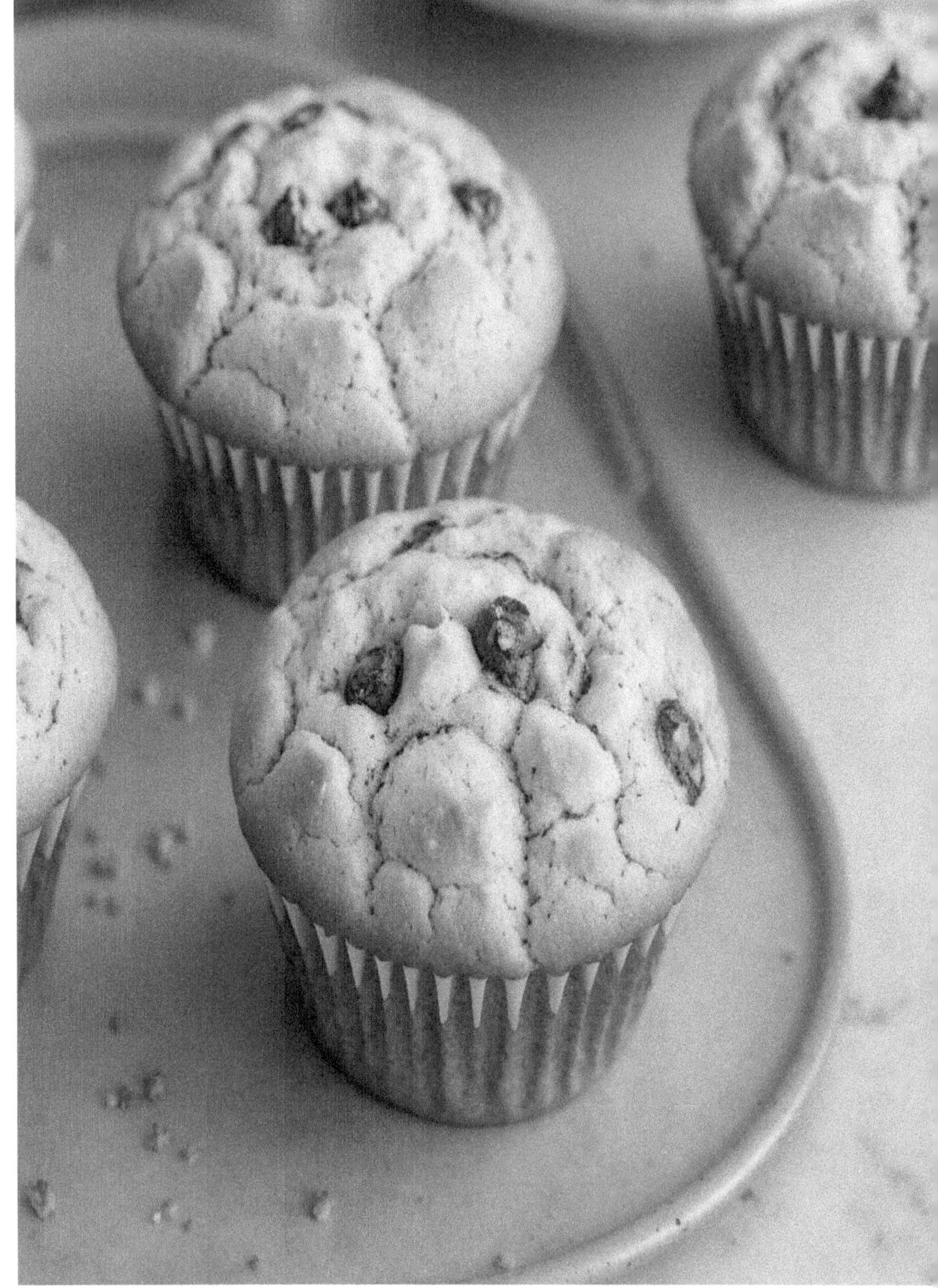

Chapter Five
Sweet Treats Naturally: Indulge Your Sweet Tooth Without Guilt

Ditch the processed sugar and artificial flavors! This chapter is your guide to creating delicious and guilt-free desserts using wholesome ingredients. We'll explore naturally sweet fruits, nuts, seeds, and spices to satisfy your cravings without compromising your health.

1. Baked Apples with Spiced Oat Crumble:

These baked apples are a classic comfort dessert with a healthy twist. Warm, tender apples are topped with a satisfying oat crumble made with rolled oats, nuts, and warming spices.

Ingredients:
- 4 apples (such as Granny Smith, Honeycrisp, or a mix)
- 1/4 cup rolled oats
- 2 tablespoons chopped walnuts or pecans
- 1 tablespoon ground cinnamon
- 1/4 teaspoon ground nutmeg
- 1/4 cup chopped pitted dates
- 2 tablespoons melted coconut oil

Method:
- Preheat oven to 375°F (190°C).
- Lightly grease a baking dish.
- Core the apples, leaving the bottom intact. You can remove a little more flesh to create a larger cavity for the filling.
- In a medium bowl, combine rolled oats, chopped nuts, cinnamon, nutmeg, and chopped dates.

> Pour in the melted coconut oil and mix until everything is well coated and crumbly.
> Fill the apple cores with the oat crumble mixture. Place the stuffed apples in the prepared baking dish.
> Bake for 30-35 minutes, or until the apples are tender and the crumble topping is golden brown.

Serving Suggestion:
> Serve the baked apples with spiced oat crumble warm or at room temperature.
> Top with a dollop of coconut yogurt or unsweetened applesauce for an extra creamy touch.

2. Vegan Chocolate Avocado Mousse:

This decadent mousse is surprisingly healthy and vegan! Creamy avocado and ripe bananas create a luxurious texture, while cocoa powder adds a rich chocolatey flavor.

Ingredients:
> 2 ripe avocados, pitted and peeled
> 2 ripe bananas, frozen and chopped
> 1/3 cup unsweetened cocoa powder
> 2 tablespoons maple syrup
> 1 teaspoon vanilla extract
> Pinch of salt

Method:
> In a high-powered blender, combine the avocados, frozen bananas, cocoa powder, maple syrup, vanilla extract, and salt.
> Blend until smooth and creamy, scraping down the sides as needed.

Finishing Touches:
> Taste and adjust sweetness with additional maple syrup if desired.

Serving Suggestion:

- ➤ Divide the vegan chocolate avocado mousse into individua serving cups or bowls.
- ➤ Chill in the refrigerator for at least 30 minutes before serving.
- ➤ Garnish with fresh berries, chopped nuts, or a drizzle of meltec dark chocolate (optional).

3. Blueberry Crisp with Almond Flour Topping:

This vibrant fruit crisp features juicy blueberries bursting witl flavor, nestled under a crumbly and delicious almond flou topping.

Ingredients:

- ➤ For the Fruit Filling:
- ➤ 4 cups fresh blueberries
- ➤ 1/4 cup cornstarch
- ➤ 2 tablespoons lemon juice
- ➤ 1/4 cup maple syrup
- ➤ 1/4 teaspoon ground cinnamon
- ➤ For the Almond Flour Topping:
- ➤ 1/2 cup almond flour
- ➤ 1/4 cup rolled oats
- ➤ 2 tablespoons chopped pecans
- ➤ 2 tablespoons melted coconut oil
- ➤ 1/4 teaspoon ground cinnamon
- ➤ Pinch of salt

Method (for the Fruit Filling):

- ➤ In a large bowl, combine blueberries, cornstarch, lemor juice, maple syrup, and ground cinnamon.
- ➤ Toss gently to coat the berries evenly.
- ➤ Preheat oven to 375°F (190°C). Pour the blueberry mixture into a greased baking dish.

Method (for the Almond Flour Topping):
- In a medium bowl, combine almond flour, rolled oats, chopped pecans, melted coconut oil, ground cinnamon, and salt.
- Mix until crumbly.

Assembling the Crisp:
- Sprinkle the almond flour topping evenly over the blueberry filling in the baking dish.

Baking:
- Bake for 40-45 minutes, or until the fruit filling is bubbling and the topping is golden brown.

Serving Suggestion:
- Serve the blueberry crisp with almond flour topping warm or at room temperature.
- Enjoy it on its own or with a scoop of vanilla ice cream (optional) for an extra treat.

4. Naturally Sweetened Carrot Cake Cookies with Cream Cheese Frosting:

These soft and chewy cookies are bursting with carrot flavor and studded with chopped nuts and raisins. A creamy vegan cream cheese frosting takes them over the top!

Ingredients:
- For the Cookies:
- 1 1/2 cups all-purpose flour
- 1 teaspoon baking soda
- 1 teaspoon ground cinnamon
- 1/2 teaspoon ground nutmeg
- 1/4 teaspoon salt
- 1 cup unsweetened applesauce
- 1/2 cup melted coconut oil
- 1/2 cup granulated sugar

- ➢ 1/4 cup packed light brown sugar
- ➢ 2 large eggs (flaxseed egg substitute for vegan option)
- ➢ 1 teaspoon vanilla extract
- ➢ 1 cup grated carrots
- ➢ 1/2 cup chopped walnuts or pecans
- ➢ 1/2 cup raisins
- ➢ For the Vegan Cream Cheese Frosting:
- ➢ 1/2 cup vegan cream cheese, softened
- ➢ 1/4 cup powdered sugar
- ➢ 1 tablespoon maple syrup
- ➢ 1 teaspoon vanilla extract
- ➢ Pinch of salt

Method (for the Cookies):

- ➢ Preheat oven to 375°F (190°C).
- ➢ Line baking sheets with parchment paper.
- ➢ In a medium bowl, whisk together flour, baking soda, cinnamon, nutmeg, and salt.
- ➢ In a large bowl, whisk together applesauce, melted coconut oil, granulated sugar, and brown sugar.
- ➢ Beat in the eggs (or flaxseed egg substitute) one at a time, then stir in vanilla extract.
- ➢ Gradually add the dry ingredients to the wet ingredients, mixing until just combined. Fold in the grated carrots, chopped nuts, and raisins.

Baking the Cookies:

- ➢ Drop rounded tablespoons of dough onto the prepared baking sheets, leaving space between each cookie for spreading.

- ➢ Bake for 10-12 minutes, or until the edges are golden brown and the centers are set.

Method (for the Vegan Cream Cheese Frosting):

> In a small bowl, cream together vegan cream cheese, powdered sugar, maple syrup, vanilla extract, and salt until smooth and spreadable.

Finishing Touches:
> Allow the cookies to cool completely on the baking sheets before frosting.
> Spread a dollop of frosting on top of each cooled cookie.

Serving Suggestion:
> Enjoy the naturally sweetened carrot cake cookies with vegan cream cheese frosting as a delicious and wholesome dessert or a satisfying afternoon snack.

5. No-Bake Vegan Chocolate Energy Balls:

These energy balls are packed with healthy fats, fiber, and natural sweetness, making them a perfect pick-me-up or satisfying snack. They're also completely vegan and require no baking!

Ingredients:
> 1 cup rolled oats
> 1/2 cup chopped nuts (such as almonds, peanuts, or cashews)
> 1/2 cup pitted Medjool dates
> 1/4 cup unsweetened shredded coconut
> 2 tablespoons cocoa powder
> 1/4 cup nut butter (such as almond butter or peanut butter)
> 2 tablespoons chia seeds (optional)
> Pinch of salt

Method:
> In a food processor, pulse the rolled oats and chopped nuts until they become a coarse flour consistency.
> Add the pitted Medjool dates, shredded coconut, cocoa powder, nut butter, chia seeds (if using), and salt.

> Process until the mixture comes together and forms a sticky dough.

Shaping the Balls:
> With wet or oiled hands, roll the mixture into tablespoon-sized balls.

Serving Suggestion:
> Store the no-bake vegan chocolate energy balls in an airtight container in the refrigerator for up to a week.
> Enjoy them as a pre-workout snack, a healthy dessert option, or a satisfying afternoon pick-me-up.

6. Roasted Spiced Pears with Vanilla Cashew Cream:

This elegant dessert features roasted pears infused with warm spices, served with a creamy and decadent cashew cream. It's a simple yet impressive treat that highlights seasonal flavors.

Ingredients:
> 4 ripe pears (such as Bosc or Bartlett)
> 1 tablespoon melted coconut oil
> 1/2 teaspoon ground cinnamon
> 1/4 teaspoon ground nutmeg
> Pinch of ground cloves
> For the Vanilla Cashew Cream:
> 1 cup raw cashews, soaked for at least 4 hours or overnight
> 1/2 cup water
> 2 tablespoons maple syrup
> 1 teaspoon vanilla extract
> Pinch of ground cinnamon

Method (for Roasting Pears):
> Preheat oven to 375°F (190°C).

- ➢ Line a baking sheet with parchment paper.
- ➢ Halve the pears lengthwise and core them. Brush the cut sides of the pears with melted coconut oil.
- ➢ In a small bowl, combine ground cinnamon, nutmeg, and cloves.
- ➢ Sprinkle the spice mixture evenly over the cut sides of the pears.

Roasting:

- ➢ Place the pears on the prepared baking sheet, cut side down. Roast for 20-25 minutes, or until the pears are tender and slightly golden brown.

Method (for Vanilla Cashew Cream):

- ➢ Drain the soaked cashews and rinse them thoroughly. In a high-powered blender, combine the cashews, water, maple syrup, vanilla extract, and ground cinnamon.
- ➢ Blend until smooth and creamy, scraping down the sides as needed.

Serving Suggestion:

- ➢ Serve the roasted spiced pears warm or at room temperature, drizzled with the vanilla cashew cream.

7. **Tropical Fruit Salad with Coconut Lime Dressing:**

This refreshing and vibrant salad showcases a variety of tropical fruits, tossed in a light and flavorful coconut lime dressing. It's a perfect way to satisfy your sweet tooth while keeping things cool and healthy.

Ingredients:

- ➢ 2 cups mixed tropical fruits (such as mango, pineapple, papaya, kiwi)
- ➢ 1/4 cup chopped fresh mint

- ➤ For the Coconut Lime Dressing:
- ➤ 1/4 cup unsweetened coconut milk
- ➤ 2 tablespoons lime juice
- ➤ 1 tablespoon honey
- ➤ 1 teaspoon grated ginger

Method (for the Dressing):

- ➤ In a small bowl, whisk together unsweetened coconut milk lime juice, honey, and grated ginger.

Assembling the Salad:

- ➤ In a large bowl, combine the mixed tropical fruits and chopped fresh mint.

Adding the Dressing:

- ➤ Pour the coconut lime dressing over the fruit salad and toss gently to coat everything evenly.

Serving Suggestion:

- ➤ Serve the tropical fruit salad with coconut lime dressing chilled for maximum refreshment. It's a light and healthy dessert option or a perfect side dish for a summer meal.

8. Vegan Chocolate Chip Cookie Bars:

These chewy and delicious cookie bars are packed with vegan chocolate chips and can be made gluten-free with a simple substitution.

Ingredients:

- ➤ 1 ½ cups all-purpose flour (or gluten-free flour blend for gluten-free option)
- ➤ 1/2 teaspoon baking soda
- ➤ 1/4 teaspoon salt
- ➤ 1/2 cup vegan butter, softened
- ➤ 3/4 cup packed light brown sugar

- ➢ 1/4 cup granulated sugar
- ➢ 1 tablespoon flaxseed meal (mixed with 3 tablespoons water for egg replacement)
- ➢ 1 teaspoon vanilla extract
- ➢ 1 cup vegan chocolate chips

Method:

- ➢ Preheat oven to 350°F (175°C).
- ➢ Line a 9x13 inch baking pan with parchment paper.
- ➢ In a medium bowl, whisk together flour (or gluten-free flour blend) and baking soda.
- ➢ In a large bowl, cream together vegan butter, brown sugar, and granulated sugar until light and fluffy. Beat in the flaxseed egg mixture (or regular egg if not vegan) and vanilla extract.
- ➢ Gradually add the dry ingredients to the wet ingredients, mixing until just combined. Fold in the vegan chocolate chips.

Baking the Bars:

- ➢ Pour the batter into the prepared baking pan and spread evenly.
- ➢ Bake for 20-25 minutes, or until the edges are golden brown and the center is set but still slightly soft.

Cooling and Cutting:

- ➢ Let the cookie bars cool completely in the pan on a wire rack before cutting.
- ➢ Once cool, cut into squares or bars for serving.

Serving Suggestion:

- ➢ Enjoy the vegan chocolate chip cookie bars warm from the oven with a glass of plant-based milk, or store them in an airtight container at room temperature for up to 3 days.

9. Strawberry Chia Seed Jam with Almond Butter Toast:

This breakfast or snack option is surprisingly sweet and satisfying. Chia seeds create a delicious jam-like texture, while almond butter adds a creamy richness.

Ingredients:
- For the Strawberry Chia Seed Jam:
- 1 cup fresh or frozen strawberries
- 1/4 cup chia seeds
- 1/4 cup maple syrup
- 1 tablespoon lemon juice
- For the Toast:
- 2 slices whole-wheat bread
- 2 tablespoons almond butter

Method (for the Strawberry Chia Seed Jam):
- In a small saucepan, combine fresh or frozen strawberries, chia seeds, maple syrup, and lemon juice.
- Heat over medium heat, stirring occasionally, until the mixture thickens and becomes jam-like, about 5-7 minutes.
- Remove from heat and let cool slightly. The jam will thicken further as it cools.

Assembling the Toast:
- Toast the whole-wheat bread slices to your desired level of doneness.
- Spread almond butter evenly on each slice of toast.
- Top the almond butter toast with a generous dollop of strawberry chia seed jam.

Serving Suggestion:
- Enjoy the strawberry chia seed jam with almond butter toast as a nutritious and satisfying breakfast or a delightful afternoon snack.

10. Dark Chocolate Dipped Banana Bites with Toasted Coconut Flakes:

This simple yet decadent treat features fresh banana slices dipped in melted dark chocolate and then rolled in toasted coconut flakes. It's a fun and healthy alternative to candy-coated treats.

Ingredients:
- 2 ripe bananas, sliced into bite-sized pieces
- 1/2 cup dark chocolate chips (at least 60% cacao)
- 1/4 cup unsweetened shredded coconut flakes

Method:
- Prepare a baking sheet lined with parchment paper.
- In a small heatproof bowl, melt the dark chocolate chips using a double boiler method or short microwave bursts with stirring until smooth.
- Toast the shredded coconut flakes in a dry skillet over medium heat, stirring frequently, until golden brown. Be careful not to burn the flakes.

Dipping and Coating:
- Using a fork or tongs, dip each banana slice into the melted dark chocolate, coating it completely.
- Immediately transfer the chocolate-dipped banana slice to the prepared baking sheet.
- Sprinkle the top of the coated banana slice with toasted coconut flakes.

Refrigerate and Serve:
- Place the baking sheet with chocolate-dipped banana bites in the refrigerator for at least 30 minutes, or until the chocolate is set.

Serving Suggestion:
- Enjoy the dark chocolate dipped banana bites with toasted coconut flakes as a delicious and healthy dessert or a satisfying sweet snack.

> Store leftover bites in an airtight container in the refrigerator for
  up to 3 days.

11. Spiced Sweet Potato Stacks with Walnut Crumble:

These layered treats are a delightful combination of creamy sweet
potato puree, warming spices, and a crunchy walnut crumble
topping. They're naturally gluten-free and perfect for a satisfying
and healthy dessert.

Ingredients:
> For the Sweet Potato Filling:
> 2 medium sweet potatoes, peeled and diced
> 1/4 cup water
> 1/4 cup unsweetened coconut milk
> 1/2 teaspoon ground cinnamon
> 1/4 teaspoon ground nutmeg
> Pinch of ground ginger
> 1 tablespoon maple syrup
> For the Walnut Crumble:
> 1/2 cup chopped walnuts
> 1/4 cup rolled oats (use gluten-free oats for gluten-free
  option)
> 2 tablespoons chopped pitted dates
> 1 tablespoon melted coconut oil
> 1/4 teaspoon ground cinnamon

Method (for the Sweet Potato Filling):
> In a medium saucepan, combine diced sweet potatoes,
  water, coconut milk, cinnamon, nutmeg, ginger, and maple
  syrup.

> Bring to a boil, then reduce heat and simmer for 15-20 minutes, or until the sweet potatoes are tender and can be easily mashed.
> Using a potato masher or immersion blender, mash the sweet potatoes until smooth. Set aside.

Method (for the Walnut Crumble):

> Preheat oven to 375°F (190°C).
> In a small bowl, combine chopped walnuts, rolled oats, chopped dates, melted coconut oil, and ground cinnamon.
> Mix until crumbly.

Assembling the Stacks:

> Divide the sweet potato puree evenly between two ramekins or small baking dishes.
> Sprinkle the walnut crumble topping over the sweet potato puree in each dish.

Baking:

> Bake for 15-20 minutes, or until the crumble topping is golden brown and the sweet potato filling is heated through.

Serving Suggestion:

> Serve the spiced sweet potato stacks with walnut crumble warm or at room temperature.
> Enjoy them on their own or with a dollop of whipped coconut cream for an extra decadent touch.

12. Gluten-Free Vegan Brownies with Black Bean Surprise:

These brownies are fudgy, delicious, and secretly packed with black beans! They're gluten-free, vegan, and a great way to sneak in some extra nutrients without compromising on flavor.

Ingredients:

> 1 can (15 oz) black beans, rinsed and drained
> 1/2 cup rolled oats (use certified gluten-free oats for gluten free option)
> 1/4 cup unsweetened cocoa powder
> 1/4 cup chopped walnuts or pecans
> 1/4 cup pitted Medjool dates
> 2 tablespoons melted coconut oil
> 1 teaspoon vanilla extract
> Pinch of salt

Method:
> Preheat oven to 350°F (175°C).
> Line an 8x8 inch baking pan with parchment paper.
> In a food processor, combine rinsed and drained black beans, rolled oats, cocoa powder, chopped nuts, pitted dates, melted coconut oil, vanilla extract, and salt.
> Process until a thick and sticky batter forms.

Baking the Brownies:
> Pour the batter into the prepared baking pan and spread evenly. Bake for 20-25 minutes, or until a toothpick inserted into the center comes out with moist crumbs (not completely clean).

Cooling and Cutting:
> Let the brownies cool completely in the pan on a wire rack before cutting.
> Once cool, cut into squares for serving.

Serving Suggestion:
> Enjoy the gluten-free vegan brownies with black bean surprise as a satisfying and healthy dessert option.

> Store leftover brownies in an airtight container at room temperature for up to 3 days.

12. Homemade Applesauce with Spiced Walnuts:

This simple recipe transforms apples into a naturally sweet and flavorful applesauce. Toasted walnuts with a hint of spice add a delightful textural and taste contrast.

Ingredients:
> 4 medium apples (such as Granny Smith, Honeycrisp, or a mix)
> 1/4 cup water
> 1/4 teaspoon ground cinnamon
> 1/4 teaspoon ground nutmeg
> Pinch of ground cloves
> For the Spiced Walnuts:
> 1/4 cup chopped walnuts
> 1/2 teaspoon ground cinnamon
> Pinch of ground ginger

Method (for the Applesauce):
> Peel, core, and chop the apples into bite-sized pieces.
> In a medium saucepan, combine chopped apples, water, cinnamon, nutmeg, and cloves.
> Bring to a boil, then reduce heat and simmer for 15-20 minutes, or until the apples are tender and softened.
> Using a potato masher or immersion blender, mash the apples to your desired consistency.
> You can leave it chunky for a more rustic texture or mash it smoother for a creamier applesauce.

Method (for the Spiced Walnuts):

- In a small skillet over medium heat, toast the chopped walnuts until fragrant and slightly golden brown, stirring frequently to avoid burning.
- Remove the toasted walnuts from the heat and sprinkle with ground cinnamon and ginger.
- Toss to coat the walnuts evenly with the spices.

Serving Suggestion:
- Serve the homemade applesauce warm or chilled.
- Top with a sprinkle of the spiced walnuts for a delicious and satisfying snack or a healthy dessert option.
- You can also enjoy the applesauce with a dollop of plain yogurt or whipped cream for an extra touch of creaminess.

13. No-Bake Vegan Raspberry Chia Seed Pudding:

This vibrant and refreshing pudding is perfect for a light and healthy dessert. Layers of creamy chia seed pudding and tart raspberries create a delightful flavor and texture combination.

Ingredients:
- 1 cup unsweetened plant-based milk (such as almond milk or coconut milk)
- 1/4 cup chia seeds
- 1/4 cup fresh or frozen raspberries
- 1 tablespoon maple syrup
- 1/2 teaspoon vanilla extract

For garnish (optional):
- Fresh raspberries
- Mint leaves

Method:

- ➢ In a small jar or container, combine unsweetened plant-based milk, chia seeds, maple syrup, and vanilla extract. Stir well to combine.
- ➢ Gently fold in half of the raspberries.

Refrigeration:
- ➢ Cover the jar or container and refrigerate for at least 4 hours, or preferably overnight, to allow the chia seeds to absorb the liquid and thicken the pudding.

Layering and Serving:
- ➢ When ready to serve, spoon the chia seed pudding into a serving dish or individual glasses.
- ➢ Top with the remaining fresh or frozen raspberries for a beautiful layered effect.

Garnishing (optional):
- ➢ Garnish with additional fresh raspberries and mint leaves for a touch of extra color and freshness.

14. Baked Peaches with Almond Butter Drizzle and Toasted Sliced Almonds:

This simple dessert features juicy peaches baked with a touch of cinnamon, then drizzled with a decadent almond butter sauce and topped with toasted almonds.

Ingredients:
- ➢ 2 ripe peaches, halved and pitted
- ➢ 1/2 teaspoon ground cinnamon
- ➢ For the Almond Butter Drizzle:
- ➢ 1/4 cup almond butter
- ➢ 2 tablespoons maple syrup

- ➢ 1 tablespoon water
- ➢ 1/4 teaspoon vanilla extract
- ➢ For the Toasted Almonds:
- ➢ 1/4 cup sliced almonds

Method (for the Peaches):

- ➢ Preheat oven to 375°F (190°C).
- ➢ Line a baking sheet with parchment paper.
- ➢ Place the peach halves, cut side up, on the prepared baking sheet. Sprinkle the cut sides with ground cinnamon.

Baking the Peaches:

- ➢ Bake the peaches for 15-20 minutes, or until they are tender and slightly golden brown.

Method (for the Almond Butter Drizzle):

- ➢ In a small bowl, whisk together almond butter, maple syrup, water, and vanilla extract until smooth and pourable.

Method (for the Toasted Almonds):

- ➢ In a small skillet over medium heat, toast the sliced almonds until fragrant and golden brown, stirring frequently to avoid burning.

Serving Suggestion:

- ➢ Remove the baked peaches from the oven and let them cool slightly.
- ➢ Drizzle each peach half generously with the almond butter sauce.
- ➢ Sprinkle with toasted sliced almonds for added texture and flavor.
- ➢ Enjoy the baked peaches with almond butter drizzle and toasted almonds warm or at room temperature.

15. Gluten-Free Vegan Mini Cheesecakes with Berry Compote:

These creamy and decadent mini cheesecakes are surprisingly vegan and gluten-free! A delicious nut and date crust pairs perfectly with a smooth cashew cream filling, topped with a vibrant berry compote.

Ingredients:

For the Crust (use gluten-free certified oats for gluten-free option):

- 1 cup rolled oats
- 1/2 cup chopped walnuts or pecans
- 1/4 cup pitted Medjool dates
- 1/4 teaspoon ground cinnamon
- For the Cashew Cream Filling:
- 1 cup raw cashews, soaked for at least 4 hours or overnight
- 1/2 cup unsweetened coconut milk
- 2 tablespoons maple syrup
- 1 tablespoon lemon juice
- 1 teaspoon vanilla extract

For the Berry Compote:

- 1 cup mixed berries (such as strawberries, blueberries, raspberries)
- 1 tablespoon maple syrup
- 1 tablespoon cornstarch (optional, for thicker compote)

Method (for the Crust):

- In a food processor, pulse the rolled oats, chopped nuts, pitted dates, and ground cinnamon until a crumbly mixture forms.

Preparing the Muffin Tin:

- Lightly grease a 6-cup muffin tin or line it with paper liners.
- Press the prepared crust mixture evenly into the bottom of each muffin cup.

Baking the Crust (optional):

> Preheat oven to 350°F (175°C).
> Bake the crust for 10 minutes to set it slightly. This step is optional, but it can help prevent the crust from becoming soggy from the filling.
> Let the crust cool completely before adding the filling.

Method (for the Cashew Cream Filling):

> Drain the soaked cashews and rinse them thoroughly. In a high-powered blender, combine the cashews, unsweetened coconut milk, maple syrup, lemon juice, and vanilla extract. Blend until smooth and creamy, scraping down the sides as needed.

Filling the Crusts:

> Once the crusts are cool, spoon the cashew cream filling evenly into each muffin cup.

Refrigeration:

> Cover the muffin tin with plastic wrap and refrigerate for at least 4 hours, or preferably overnight, to allow the filling to set.

Method (for the Berry Compote):

> In a small saucepan, combine mixed berries and maple syrup.
> Heat over medium heat, stirring occasionally, until the berries soften and release their juices.

Optional Thickening:

> If you prefer a thicker compote, whisk together 1 tablespoon cornstarch with a little bit of water to form a slurry.

> Add the slurry to the simmering berries and cook for another minute or two, stirring constantly, until the compote thickens to your desired consistency.

Assembling and Serving:
> When ready to serve, spoon the berry compote over the chilled mini cheesecakes.

Enjoyment:
> Enjoy the gluten-free vegan mini cheesecakes with berry compote for a delicious and healthy dessert option. Store leftover cheesecakes in an airtight container in the refrigerator for up to 3 days.

17. Creamy Avocado Chocolate Mousse:

This rich and decadent mousse is surprisingly healthy! Avocados provide a creamy base, while cocoa powder and maple syrup create a delightful chocolate flavor.

Ingredients:
> 2 ripe avocados, pitted and peeled
> 1/4 cup unsweetened cocoa powder
> 1/4 cup maple syrup
> 1 tablespoon lemon juice
> 1 teaspoon vanilla extract
> Pinch of salt

For garnish (optional):
> Cocoa nibs
> Fresh mint leaves

Method:

> In a high-powered blender, combine the avocado flesh, cocoa powder, maple syrup, lemon juice, vanilla extract, and salt.
> Blend until smooth and creamy, scraping down the sides as needed.

Serving Suggestion:
> Spoon the avocado chocolate mousse into serving dishes or individual glasses.
> Garnish with optional cocoa nibs and fresh mint leaves for a touch of elegance.
> Serve the mousse chilled for a refreshing and delicious dessert.

18. Chia Seed Pudding Parfaits with Tropical Fruit and Coconut Flakes:

These layered parfaits are a fun and healthy way to enjoy chia seed pudding. Layers of creamy chia pudding, vibrant tropical fruits, and crunchy coconut flakes create a delightful textural and taste contrast.

Ingredients:
> 1 cup unsweetened plant-based milk (such as almond milk or coconut milk)
> 1/4 cup chia seeds
> 1/2 cup mixed tropical fruits (such as mango, pineapple, papaya)
> 1 tablespoon maple syrup
> 1/2 teaspoon vanilla extract
> 1/4 cup unsweetened shredded coconut flakes

Method (for the Chia Seed Pudding):

> In a small jar or container, combine unsweetened plant-based milk, chia seeds, maple syrup, and vanilla extract. Stir well to combine.

Refrigeration:
> Cover the jar or container and refrigerate for at least 4 hours, or preferably overnight, to allow the chia seeds to absorb the liquid and thicken the pudding.

Assembling the Parfaits:
> In a serving dish or individual glasses, alternate layers of chia seed pudding and mixed tropical fruits.

Adding the Crunch:
> Sprinkle each layer of fruit with unsweetened shredded coconut flakes for added texture and a touch of tropical flavor.

Serving Suggestion:
> Enjoy the chia seed pudding parfaits with tropical fruit and coconut flakes for a refreshing and healthy breakfast, snack, or light dessert.

19. Roasted Figs with Goat Cheese and Honey:

This simple yet elegant dessert features fresh figs roasted until slightly softened, then filled with a creamy goat cheese mixture and drizzled with honey.

Ingredients:
> 4 ripe figs
> 2 ounces goat cheese, softened
> 1 tablespoon honey
> Fresh thyme sprigs (for garnish, optional)

Method:

- ➢ Preheat oven to 400°F (200°C).
- ➢ Line a baking sheet with parchment paper.
- ➢ Cut the figs in half lengthwise, leaving the stem on.

Preparing the Goat Cheese Filling:

- ➢ In a small bowl, mash the softened goat cheese with a fork until smooth and creamy.

Filling the Figs:

- ➢ Spoon a dollop of the goat cheese mixture into the center of each fig half.

Baking:

- ➢ Place the fig halves, cut side up, on the prepared baking sheet.
- ➢ Bake for 10-15 minutes, or until the figs are slightly softened and the goat cheese is warmed through.

Finishing Touches:

- ➢ Drizzle each fig half with a generous amount of honey.

Serving Suggestion:

- ➢ Serve the roasted figs with goat cheese and honey warm or at room temperature.
- ➢ Garnish with fresh thyme sprigs for an extra touch of elegance, if desired. Enjoy this recipe as a delicious and sophisticated dessert option.

20. No-Bake Vegan Energy Bites with Dates, Nuts, and Cacao Nibs:

These energy bites are packed with healthy fats, fiber, and natural sweetness, making them a perfect pick-me-up or satisfying snack. They're also completely vegan and require no baking!

Ingredients:

- 1 cup pitted Medjool dates
- 1/2 cup rolled oats
- 1/4 cup chopped nuts (such as almonds, peanuts, or cashews)
- 1/4 cup unsweetened shredded coconut flakes
- 2 tablespoons chia seeds
- 2 tablespoons cacao nibs
- Pinch of salt

Method:

- In a food processor, pulse the pitted Medjool dates until they become a sticky paste.

Adding the Dry Ingredients:

- Add the rolled oats, chopped nuts, shredded coconut flakes, chia seeds, cacao nibs, and salt to the food processor.
- Process until the mixture comes together and forms a sticky dough.

Shaping the Balls:

- With wet or oiled hands, roll the mixture into tablespoon-sized balls.

Refrigeration (Optional):

- Place the energy bites in the refrigerator for at least 30 minutes to allow them to firm up. This step is optional but can help the bites hold their shape better.

Serving Suggestion:

- Store the no-bake vegan energy bites in an airtight container in the refrigerator for up to a week. Enjoy them as a pre-workout snack, a healthy dessert option, or a satisfying afternoon pick-me-up.

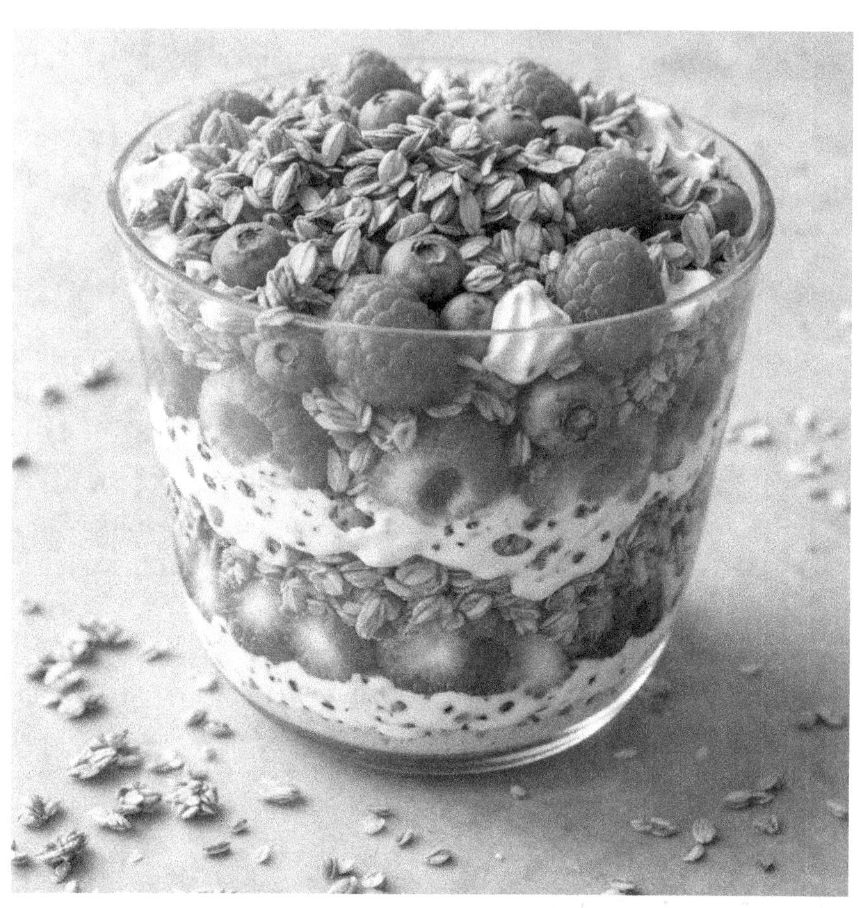

Chapter Six
Basics & Essentials - Building Your Plant-Based Kitchen

Welcome to the foundation of your plant-based culinary journey! This chapter equips you with the knowledge and skills to build a well-stocked pantry and master essential cooking techniques for a world of delicious, healthy plant-based meals.

1. Essential Pantry Staples:

Stocking your pantry with these key ingredients sets the stage for effortless plant-based cooking:

- **Whole Grains:** Brown rice, quinoa, oats, whole-wheat pasta, barley – provide sustained energy and essential nutrients.
- **Legumes:** Dried beans (kidney, pinto, black, lentils), chickpeas – versatile protein sources, rich in fiber and minerals.
- **Nuts & Seeds:** Almonds, walnuts, cashews, flaxseeds, chia seeds – healthy fats, protein, and add texture and richness.
- **Dried Fruits:** Raisins, cranberries, dates – natural sweeteners, add bursts of flavor and fiber.
- **Plant-Based Milks:** Almond milk, soy milk, coconut milk – dairy alternatives for beverages, cooking, and baking.
- **Healthy Oils:** Extra virgin olive oil, avocado oil – healthy fats for cooking and salad dressings.
- **Vinegars:** Apple cider vinegar, balsamic vinegar – add acidity and depth of flavor to sauces and dressings.
- **Spices:** Ground cumin, turmeric, paprika, chili powder, nutritional yeast – create flavor profiles and add essential vitamins.
- **Sweeteners:** Maple syrup, agave nectar, dates – natural sweeteners to replace refined sugars.
- **Canned Goods:** Diced tomatoes, chickpeas, lentils – convenient pantry staples for quick and flavorful meals.

Tip: Purchase whole grains and legumes in bulk for cost-effectiveness and less packaging waste.

2. Basic Cooking Techniques for Whole Grains & Legumes:

Mastering these techniques unlocks a world of possibilities:

Cooking Whole Grains:
- **Stovetop Method:** Simmer grains in water or broth with a pinch of salt for a simple and effective approach.
- **Rice Cooker Method:** Utilize this convenient appliance for perfect, fluffy rice every time.

Cooking Legumes:
- **Soaking:** Soaking beans overnight or for several hours helps reduce cooking time and improve digestibility.
- **Stovetop Method:** Simmer drained beans in water or broth with seasonings until tender.
- **Pressure Cooker Method:** For faster cooking times and some beans that require a longer cook time, a pressure cooker is a great option.

Tips:
- Rinse whole grains and legumes before cooking to remove debris.
- Seasoning while cooking adds depth of flavor.
- Utilize leftover cooked grains and legumes in various dishes throughout the week.

3. Creating Healthy, Delicious Sauces & Dressings:

Transform simple ingredients into flavorful sauces and dressings:

- **Creamy Lemon Herb Sauce:** Blend cashews or soaked sunflower seeds with lemon juice, nutritional yeast, garlic, and herbs for a versatile sauce for pasta, vegetables, or dipping.

- **Easy Tahini Sauce:** Combine tahini paste, lemon juice, water, garlic, and a touch of maple syrup for a flavorful sauce on salads, wraps, or bowls.
- **Roasted Tomato Marinara Sauce:** Roast tomatoes, garlic, and herbs for a naturally sweet and flavorful base for pasta dishes.
- **Balsamic Vinaigrette:** Combine olive oil, balsamic vinegar, Dijon mustard, and a pinch of salt and pepper for a classic salad dressing.
- **Peanut Sauce:** Blend peanut butter with soy sauce, rice vinegar, ginger, and a touch of maple syrup for a delicious dipping sauce for vegetables, tofu, or noodles.
- **Avocado Ranch Dressing:** Blend avocado, plant-based milk, lemon juice, garlic, herbs, and spices for a creamy and flavorful salad dressing.
- **Mango Salsa:** Combine chopped mango, red onion, cilantro, lime juice, and a touch of jalapeño (optional) for a fresh and zesty topping for tacos or bowls.
- **Ginger Sesame Dressing:** Whisk together soy sauce, rice vinegar, sesame oil, ginger, and a touch of maple syrup for a flavorful Asian-inspired dressing.
- **Cilantro Lime Crema:** Blend cashews or soaked sunflower seeds with cilantro, lime juice, garlic, and a touch of water for a bright and flavorful topping for tacos, burritos, or bowls.
- **Spicy Coconut Curry Sauce:** Sauté onions, ginger, and spices like curry powder or turmeric. Add coconut milk, vegetables, and your favorite protein source (tofu, chickpeas) for a warming and flavorful curry.

Tips:

- Experiment with different spices and herbs to create unique flavor profiles.
- Use fresh herbs whenever possible
- Use a high-powered blender or food processor to achieve a smooth and creamy consistency for sauces.

- ➢ Adjust the thickness of sauces and dressings by adding more or less water or plant-based milk.
- ➢ Taste and adjust seasonings as needed for a perfect balance of flavors.
- ➢ Store leftover sauces and dressings in airtight containers in the refrigerator for up to a week.

By mastering the basics, exploring additional options, and unleashing your creativity, you'll be well on your way to a delicious and fulfilling plant-based kitchen experience!